END YOUR COVERT MISSION

A Veteran's Guide to Fighting Pain and Addiction

Dustin Brockberg, PhD

Kerry Brockberg, PhD

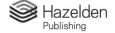
Hazelden
Publishing

Hazelden Publishing
Center City, Minnesota 55012
hazelden.org/bookstore

© 2022 by Hazelden Betty Ford Foundation
All rights reserved. Published 2022.
Printed in the United States of America

ISBN: 978-1-61649-988-4

Library of Congress Cataloging-in-Publication Data

Names: Brockberg, Dustin, author. | Brockberg, Kerry, author.
Title: End your covert mission : a veteran's guide to fighting pain and addiction / by Dustin Brockberg, PhD, LP, and Kerry Brockberg, PhD, LP.
Description: Center City, Minnesota : Hazelden Publishing, [2022] | Includes bibliographical references. | Summary: "A guide for veterans on understanding and addressing pain-including physical, emotional, and social pain-and substance use and addiction"—Provided by publisher.
Identifiers: LCCN 2022026051 (print) | LCCN 2022026052 (ebook) | ISBN 9781616499884 (paperback) | ISBN 9781616499891 (ebook)
Subjects: LCSH: Veterans—Mental health. | Veterans—Substance use. | Veterans—Health and hygiene. | Pain—Treatment.
Classification: LCC RC451.4.V48 B756 2022 (print) | LCC RC451.4.V48 (ebook) | DDC 616.890086/97—dc23/eng/20220713
LC record available at https://lccn.loc.gov/2022026051
LC ebook record available at https://lccn.loc.gov/2022026052

Editor's note

All stories shared in this book were provided with the consent of each veteran. No clinical patients were used. The names, details, and circumstances may have been changed to protect the privacy of those mentioned in this publication.

This publication is not intended as a substitute for the advice of health care professionals.

26 25 24 23 22   1 2 3 4 5 6

Cover design: Terri Kinne
Interior design and typesetting: Percolator Graphic Design
Developmental editor: Marc Olson
Editorial project manager: Cathy Broberg

"Finally—an important book centered in the veteran culture! *End Your Covert Mission* empowers the reader to draw on the strengths of the veteran experience while also acknowledging what needs to be left behind to best cope with pain in all its manifestations."

—Carey E. Gleason, PhD, MS; Madison VA GRECC and University of Wisconsin School of Medicine and Public Health

"Veterans helping veterans! This is not another outsider or academic telling veterans how they should 'feel.' This veteran couple has lived it and can help you end your covert mission!"

—Colonel Scott Jensen, U.S. Marine Corps (retired), president of Alpine Global Solutions

"As a former Army nurse and CNP with the VA for 28 years, I think this book provides a practical guide for veterans suffering from chronic pain. Having worked in pain management for 18 years, recommendations in the book are on target with the proven multidisciplinary management of chronic pain and the psychological suffering that accompanies that pain."

—Diane M. Budnick, clinical nurse practitioner

"Written from a veteran's perspective, *End Your Covert Mission* offers authentic insights and user-friendly strategies. A great resource for veterans and their loved ones wanting to live better with chronic pain."

—Paul Heideman, PhD, LP, clinical psychologist

"As an interventional pain physician, I tend to focus on the physical side of pain, but complex chronic pain is more than physical and involves psychosocial and emotional components that are equally important. I worked alongside Dr. Kerry Brockberg for several years in our multidisciplinary pain clinic where I watched her skillfully guide our patients through the maze of emotions and psychological consequences that often occur when people struggle with chronic pain. Her wonderful new book focuses on the unique circumstances of chronic pain after military service, and I believe it will help many veterans triumph over chronic pain and improve quality of life."

—David M. Schultz, MD, founder and CEO, Nura Pain Clinics, Minneapolis, MN

End Your Covert Mission

To Madison and Rylee

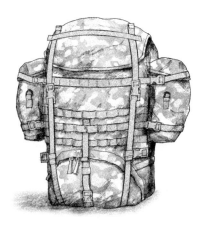

Many veterans continue to carry a ruck full of the same responses

to pain that they used in the military. It's time to empty out that

imaginary pack and upgrade your coping gear with tools and

strategies that can help you feel and function better.

CONTENTS

PREFACE

We met after Dustin got out of the Army. He served from 2004 to 2008 as a tank crewman or, in other words, a "19 Kilo" or "tanker." His service included a deployment to Iraq and a hardship tour to South Korea. In the years since we met, we've continued to learn how Dustin's time in the military influences his life, his interactions with our friends and family, and our life together as a couple.

We value the strength the military experience has brought to our relationship. We also understand that this part of Dustin's story includes pain and adds complexity to our lives. We have learned how powerful communication is for our relationship. We don't shy away from hard questions. We keep listening to each other, and we keep learning how to hear one another with empathy. This has made us closer. It has made us a team.

Along with our professional interests in pain management, rehabilitation psychology, and addiction (substance use disorder), our personal experience as a veteran couple is a big reason why we wrote this book and why we gave it the title it has. We know firsthand the value of empowering veterans to share their voice and their story, especially with pain and addiction. We believe that the mission of finding relief from pain and recovery from addiction shouldn't be covert or secret. Silence about these challenges among veterans is dangerous—both for veterans and for the people who love them. We hope our work will inspire and inform a new conversation about what pain and addiction are, how these things show up in veterans' lives, and how to cope and recover in healthy and productive ways.

We have learned a lot from the amazing veterans we've worked with over the years. Helping people like you better understand and deal with the physical, emotional, and social pain they experience—as well as the ways these different types of pain interact with and compound each other—is what we do. The success we've had in helping veterans find tangible and practical ways to manage and cope with pain that don't involve addictive substances is what drives us.

Problems with pain and addiction are challenges that can be overcome. Finding solutions often comes naturally to people with military service in their backgrounds. Veterans have been trained to manage obstacles and break complex and daunting tasks into achievable objectives. As a veteran, you have inherent strengths of character, dependability, and honor. You've accomplished more in your life already than many people ever do. These qualities and characteristics can be valuable assets in the mission of finding relief from pain and addiction.

Admitting that you have addiction problems or feel pain requires vulnerability and humility. However, mostly it requires simply being human with another person. Pain is natural. It's part of the human experience that unites us. We want veterans to know that they no longer need to hide their pain. Identifying sources of pain, sharing stories of pain, and getting help to manage pain are signs of strength and courage. The same is true when it comes to addiction—to alcohol, other drugs, or behaviors. Recovery involves being brave enough to ask for and accept support.

This book comes at a time when research, education, and training about pain and pain management have increased dramatically. We know more today about the negative impacts of not seeking help. We know how important it is to find language that accurately and honestly describes veteran pain. We know more about the negative impact of opioids and other substances, and how historically veterans have used such substances as tools to address social and emotional issues as well as to relieve physical pain. We also know more about the damage that pain and unhealthy coping strategies can do to the lives of veterans and their loved ones.

Many veterans' pain stories do not start with the traumatic experiences they faced in the military but rather have roots in trauma that occurred in childhood. Veterans may also experience traumatic events after their military service too. These realities continue to inform and shape our work.

This book is a call to action to help veterans change their mindset about pain. It will help veterans open their minds about what various types of pain look like and understand that there is no need to continue to "push through" their pain or rely on unhealthy and destructive coping strategies like concealment and substance use to manage it. There are better tools—better gear—and we are here to show you how they work.

All we ask of you for this mission is to be open, think critically, and let your voice be heard. Your voice is valuable and your pain can be shared, better understood, and transformed with the strategies we offer.

We are honored to have the opportunity to write a book for veterans that features veteran perspectives and even a veteran author. It is a privilege to be able to help bring words to what veterans may be experiencing and to help train up a cohort of people like you who decide to share their stories and change the narrative about veteran pain. We're confident that once you decide to end your covert mission and share your voice, you will be both surprised and relieved to learn that you're not alone.

ACKNOWLEDGMENTS

We want to thank our families, our veteran and military families, and our friends for their continued support while we were writing this book. We especially thank the veterans who gave us permission to share their voices in these pages. Your courage and bravery will make an impact on more veterans and those connected to veterans than you know. Your voices are powerful and inspire others to share their own voice as well!

—

Understanding the Mission

ACROSS BRANCHES OF THE MILITARY, you can find technical or field manuals for everything. Need to know how to dig a foxhole? There's a manual that can help. Need to know how to dispose of fuel in the field? A manual is waiting for you. Along with manuals, checklists, and procedure outlines, the military has developed gear for almost every possible combat and noncombat situation you can imagine.

This is a good thing. It means there is a rule book, a piece of equipment, or a step-by-step guide to any problem. In other words, every piece of gear a soldier or sailor or marine or airman needs is available, along with instructions for how to use it. But what happens when you go home to a life where there is no manual? There is not a barracks full of your buddies to shoot the shit. There is not a centralized place to get your gear or try out new tools. There are not a lot of people who understand what you went through and what you're feeling or experiencing now.

There's no field manual for being a veteran, especially a veteran who deals with pain or struggles with substance use. This book is an attempt to change that. Welcome to *End Your Covert Mission: A Veteran's Guide to Fighting Pain and Addiction.* We're here to help you end your covert pain mission—denying pain or problems with substance use, or dealing with them on your own. We also want you to understand and take on a new kind of mission—the mission of finding relief and healing from your pain as you move forward in your life beyond the military. Your challenge is to be open to new concepts related to pain, to be willing to try new strategies for managing pain in a more effective and healthy way, and to gain insight and wisdom from your own voice and your personal story of pain.

This book is for veterans, regardless of age, or gender, or how long you served, or in which branch, or if you were in combat or not, or how long you've been out. Your identity as a veteran is part of who you are as a human being. Veterans and military service members are different from civilians in lots of ways, of course, but we have a lot in common too. Being human means living in a world where pain is real and normal. That goes for veterans as well as everybody else.

We'll say that middle part again: Pain is normal. This is one of the most important things you will read in this book.

One basic mission in every life is to find relief from the pain we experience. We look for ways to endure, manage, process, understand, share, and even resolve the painful experiences that are a part of our life story. As with any mission, there are good and effective ways of doing this, and there are also dangerous, shortsighted, lonely, and destructive ways. As a veteran, you've probably tried a few of each.

The good news is that this world is full of healing and help. It's a world of power and possibility. We live in a world of connections, care, relaxation, and rest. That's what we hope this book can offer you. We're here to help you get briefed on the mission of living in a world where pain is real and present every day—and where you can do something about it. We're also here to help you get equipped for this mission with solid information, the best possible gear, and tons of support and encouragement.

You're already on this mission, of course. You've been on it since the day you were born. Your life has included training, lessons, and experiences that have taught you what pain is and ways to deal with it. This included your life before the military as well as what you picked up during your time of military service and what came after. All that training has sunk in and helped you get to wherever you are today.

Our guess is that you're reading this book because the tools and strategies you're currently using for dealing with pain don't feel as effective or helpful as they once did. It's also possible that your pain management gear has stopped working altogether—or even started to make things worse. This may especially be true if you've used or are using substances or other addictive behaviors to numb, avoid, or suppress your pain.

We can work with that.

In addition to identifying some of the unhelpful and unhealthy ways you may be managing your pain, this book outlines the benefits of finding alternative healthy coping strategies for dealing with pain over the longer term. It offers practical, effective tools that you can start using today. Some of the Tangible Next Steps at the end of each chapter are exercises or tasks that you can add to your toolkit right away, some are suggestions for things you can try when you have the opportunity, and some are invitations to shift your mind into a different way of thinking. Sometimes we'll challenge you to move beyond your comfort zone when you feel ready and able. Many veterans are already on this path. We'll feature some of their voices in each chapter.

Some of the stories you'll hear from veterans may resonate with your experience, and maybe some will touch painful memories. You may need to read this book at your own pace, or even skip parts of it you don't feel ready to read. You'll also hear from veterans who have found ways to open up and share. Trust their lead and consider following their example. We're grateful for all the veterans who shared their stories.

Keeping pain covert is not something you learned overnight. At some point in the past, not letting someone know you were vulnerable or hurting may have helped you survive or endure. That's understandable. What we know today is that this strategy is not helpful for the long haul. Whatever emotions or experiences you've hidden or bottled up don't need to be held on to or concealed for years and years to come.

Secrets and silence keep us stuck and sick. It is time to get unstuck and start feeling better. It's time to tackle your pain by speaking up and speaking out, or just talking one-on-one with somebody who cares. We are here to guide you. We're going to give you gear and support for finding relief from pain in ways that respect who you are and fit what you want from life.

How to Use This Book

As you read the following chapters, you'll notice a few recurring elements that go along with the information and encouragement we've presented.

Veteran Voices

We asked a bunch of veterans to help us tell the story that became this book. Many of their voices appear along the way, often at the start of chapters. These are people who have experienced many of the same things that you're dealing with. They've endured pain and suffered loss. Some have struggled to find coping gear that helps them find relief from the pain that veteran life may involve. Others are battling addiction. These veterans shared their stories because they want to help their brothers and sisters—that's you. And you've got your own story to tell and your own wisdom to explore. At the end of the book, you'll find a set of prompts that can help you share your unique veteran voice to end the covert mission of silent suffering.

Checkpoint Questions

These questions are intended to get you thinking about your current ideas and behavior when it comes to managing pain and addiction. We hope you'll take the time to reflect and answer these questions. You can do this in your head, or keep a journal, or make a voice memo on your phone. You can also use Checkpoint questions to start conversations with others about what you're thinking and feeling. This might include other veterans or close friends, family members, or health care providers.

Tangible Next Steps

Each chapter closes with a collection of practical tools—ways you can start to find new pain management gear or improve the gear you already use.

Some steps ask you to try thinking differently right away. They challenge you to experiment with new ideas, mindsets, and attitudes. Often these are the steps you need to take before anything else stands a chance of success. Don't discount the power of changing your thoughts. Doing so can change your whole world.

Other steps invite you to take action. Sometimes this will mean picking up a pencil and writing a list. Sometimes it will include trying an exercise or focusing on how your body feels or what your senses are telling you. These steps are intended to be taken immediately.

A few steps challenge you to apply ideas or suggestions the next time you have an opportunity or in the future. Changing your approach to managing or coping with pain includes trying new ways of being in the world, especially when it comes to interacting with other people or unknown situations. These are the steps that can help you practice with the gear we're offering. Some of these steps take time to try out, and some steps will take multiple tries to see what works best for you.

CHAPTER ONE

—

The Mission Brief

> *All of us need help in one form or another, and most of us want help, but at our own pace and under our own terms. Most of us know that our coping mechanisms are harmful to ourselves and our families, but oftentimes we feel that "this is all I have."*
>
> —JIM, US ARMY

ENDING THE COVERT quality of your pain mission and beginning a new, shared mission of dealing with pain with honesty and courage is what this journey—and this book—is all about. In the pages that follow you'll find multiple tools and strategies that are guided by a few core beliefs. You'll probably get tired of hearing us repeat them, but they're important. Here's our bias: The most unhelpful strategy for dealing with any kind of pain is to deny it or pretend it isn't happening. The second most unhelpful strategy is keeping it to yourself or secret. The mission of experiencing, enduring, managing, and healing from pain is not supposed to be covert. The most helpful and successful ways to find sustainable, ongoing relief from pain involve sharing your burden with other people and accepting outside help from people and providers you can trust.

Human beings are meant to be in communities of relationship and mutual support. The military knows this; it's why they put soldiers into units and squads. This is where we function at our best, and where we're best able to give and receive help and care—gifts that can make any experience more bearable. This is true for active military members and it's true for veterans too.

We didn't ask for pain. Pain is part of the universal human experience. However, because we all experience pain differently, everybody's pain-relief mission is unique to them, even when there are similarities. This book focuses on the multiple types of pain veterans experience—including the pain and problems that come with addiction. In many cases, your military background has made the mission you face more difficult than it is for people who have not served.

As we'll explore in the next chapter, veterans often deal with more pain, more intense pain, and more interrelated types of pain than is typical in the civilian population. And even though they turned in the physical gear the government issued them, many veterans continue to carry a ruck full of military responses to all this pain. It's time to empty out that imaginary pack and upgrade your pain management and coping gear with tools and techniques that can help you feel and function better.

This chapter begins with a look at the various ways pain shows up in our lives, why it exists at all, and why it can be so hard to describe or define. We'll ask you to take a shot at putting words to your own experiences with pain, and we'll discuss some of the most common unhelpful strategies veterans use to deal with pain. The chapter closes with a big-picture look at what healthy coping looks like and describes how a new approach to pain—with a different set of tools—can make a difference in your life.

There's More Than One Kind of Pain

Across cultures and throughout history, people have endured and struggled with the reality of pain. Everybody hurts. We have different tolerances for how much pain we're able to bear and different ways of describing or evaluating what hurts and what to do with it. But there's a basic understanding that being alive in this world includes all kinds of discomfort. Pain can come from physical injuries and illness. We also feel pain and suffering when we lose things that are important to us or when we experience conflict, isolation, or breaks in our relationships with other people.

In this guide, we'll describe and discuss three categories of pain that are common among veterans: physical pain, emotional pain, and social pain. Each category gets its own chapter. We'll discuss what makes each type of pain distinct and talk about how they interact with one another.

This idea that there are multiple types of pain isn't new. Research into how people experience pain and the best ways to treat and relieve it has demonstrated the importance of viewing pain from what's known as a "biopsychosocial" perspective. This means that whenever we talk about pain, we need to take the following into account:

- the biology of the physical being (*bio*)
- the psychological impact of the person's life experiences (*psycho*)
- the many relationships and interactions that the person has with the environment and the people around them (*social*)

Even though this concept isn't new, not everybody gets it at first. Most people identify obvious physical pain as "pain." They don't always think about emotional and social factors that influence our experience of physical discomfort and that can be sources of pain in their own right. It becomes easier to understand if we stop and listen to the way people talk. Losing a battle buddy "hurts like hell." Feeling excluded or judged unfairly "stings." Getting a divorce can leave us "feeling gutted." Even less dramatic experiences like transitioning from military to civilian jobs or re-engaging with friends you haven't seen for years often get described with terms like "uncomfortable" or "hard" or "heavy." Pain is a reality that includes our thoughts and feelings and memories as well as physical sensations.

If the biopsychosocial idea of pain is a new one for you, welcome to it. We hope this model can help you understand the varied dimensions of pain you may be experiencing—even if you haven't had words for it before.

In chapter 3, on physical pain, we'll explain a little more about the mind and body processes that are going on whenever we experience pain of any type. Later chapters will explore veterans' experiences with emotional and social pain as well as the way addictive substances and behaviors can complicate every kind of pain.

For now, it's enough to note that your experience of physical pain often comes with emotional pain like distress or worry, and even social pain if your injury or physical condition isolates you from others. It goes the other way, too. If you've ever gotten a stomachache after being rejected or judged or felt a headache coming on when you were anxious about something, you've experienced the connection between social, emotional, and physical pain.

You may ask yourself, *Did my physical pain make me feel emotional or disconnected?* or *Did I feel disconnected and now my pain feels worse?* We can explore the "Did the chicken come before the egg or the egg before the chicken?" question all day. It's enough to know that all your experiences of pain can legitimately be called pain, they're all real, they're all related, and each type of pain can be managed, coped with, and sometimes even resolved.

CHECKPOINT:

- What experiences or feelings come to mind first when you consider the word "pain"?
- When in your life have you experienced overlaps between the pain types described above (physical, emotional, and social)?

Why Do We Hurt at All?

We actually need pain. Maybe you just said, *What!?* Stick with us. Imagine if you didn't experience pain. Imagine not noticing where the limits or edges of your physical self were. Your body wouldn't know when to stop pushing itself. Your mind wouldn't have a set of criteria for assessing danger or safety. If you've ever accidentally bit your cheek or tongue after a dental visit because your mouth was numb, you have an idea what this might be like.

On the emotional and social side, pain helps us know what's important. A life without emotional pain wouldn't allow us to experience a great deal of happiness. Our ability to endure pain and challenges provides context and contrast for feelings of success and satisfaction. If we didn't experience the pain that comes from tension or conflict in important relationships, we'd have a hard time growing and knowing what it means to be well connected to others.

Don't get us wrong. Even though we're pointing out why pain exists and what makes it a useful and even a valuable part of human existence, we won't be providing tips for how to keep feeling pain. Experiencing pain sucks. Yet understanding why it exists in the first place and what makes painful experiences an inescapable part of being human may offer some relief. Knowing that pain is normal also means that sharing your pain with others doesn't have to be scary or feel weird. Recognizing that everyone else experiences pain helps us relate to and connect with the people around us.

Pain Is Both a Function and a Feeling

As we noted above, pain is part of the body's system of self-protection. Pain sensations are intended to provide urgent information to the thinking parts of our brains. When we feel pain, it's like a sensor is going off warning us that something is going wrong or that something already wrong is about to be worse.

That said, most people don't first think of pain as a biological function. We usually think of pain as physical sensations and feelings. We know what hurts and we try to put that feeling into words by describing how something hurts and how bad. Most of us learned how to talk about pain early in our lives, progressing from simple words like "owie" or "boo-boo" to more specific and mature terms. Even as our vocabularies get bigger as grown-ups, we don't always know how best to talk about or precisely describe what we're feeling. Finding ways to help others understand our internal experience means learning and experimenting with new pain language.

Pain can be felt and described as broad and general or localized. It can be sharp or dull or prickly or searing. We might use words like "ache" or "sting" or "burn" to talk about how we feel. Sound like a lot of options? It is. Pain is something that happens on a spectrum. And it can be difficult to define or pin down these experiences and sensations. Hell, one of the most common ways medical professionals try to understand the severity of someone's pain is by asking them to rate it on a scale of 1–10. In general, pain is often hard to define and describe to others.

Although we each experience pain differently and describe it with different words (or numbers), one thing we can all typically agree on is that pain is uncomfortable and undesirable. When most people hear the word, they don't picture something happy. Pain is something we want to get rid of, or make stop, or move past.

How Do You Describe Pain?
—

We're about to challenge you to come up with your own personal description of the pain you're experiencing or have experienced.

Let's start with a list of adjectives and other descriptive words. Circle the words that make the most sense in describing your pain.

Hurt	Unhealthy	Injury
Burn	Aching	Misunderstood
Irritation	Sadness	Necessary evil
Anxious	Suffering	Loss
Angry	Uncomfortable	Dealing with
Enduring	Disconnected	Cramping
Bothersome	Sore	Challenging
Unmanageable	Sharp	Unbearable
Disconnected	Dull	Impossible

Other: _____

Other: _____

Other: _____

Now grab a piece of paper and write a one- or two-sentence definition of pain, or a statement about pain, that uses some or all of the words you circled. If you don't want to write, do this in your head. Come up with a couple of true statements that explain, describe, or define your pain. When you're done, save this paper or make a note on your phone. As you continue to use this book, you may want to revisit what you've written and make changes, additions, or deletions. You may want to expand it into a paragraph or even a letter. You may even decide to share it with someone else.

Finding ways to define and describe the types and qualities of our pain can help us get us get clarity about what we're feeling (or not feeling). It can help us better understand our own subjective experiences with pain. The act of putting words to our pain may also reveal our attitude when it comes to pain or ways we might be judging, discounting, or avoiding pain. We might also pick up some clues for ways to address or deal with our pain. Once we know what they are, we stand a chance of learning to influence our feelings and make choices about how we want to respond to them. This can also be a first step toward sharing our experience of pain with others.

Pain Affects Our Perception

Defining pain, or even circling words that best describe your experience, may have been challenging for you. Each of us carries memories of unique painful experiences that influence the way we think and talk about pain. You may not have found the words you needed in the short list of options we provided. Perhaps talking about pain hasn't ever seemed like an option for you, so finding words for it hasn't been necessary. Maybe you're just out of practice. That's okay! Remember, you're learning to use some new-to-you tools.

Part of what makes pain so hard to put words to is the way our brains work. Our thoughts about pain are connected to and filtered by our painful experiences—especially ongoing or chronic pain.

One of the brain's strengths is its ability to make associations. Associations are like shortcuts. They're pathways of thought that allow our brains to link our current experiences with previous ones. The strongest associations are often negative. Like a pain response, this is part of the way our minds try to protect us and keep us alert for any signs of a negative experience. This could be a word, a sound, a smell, or a sensation—even an activity. Even if the thing we're experiencing at the moment isn't painful or scary, we may feel a connection to the prior memory of pain. These associations, which link past experience with what we perceive in the present, can lead to a second brain function called generalization. Like association, generalization links two ideas together, even if linking them doesn't seem to make sense.

The image of a lens can be another helpful way to think about the daily impact of pain on perception. Imagine putting on blue-tinted eyeglasses. Whatever you looked at would be filtered by those lenses, so everything would appear as a shade of blue. This is similar to the way pain filters our outlook.

When we experience pain, we see the world differently. Ongoing pain can become part of how we interpret and interact with everything around us. This can make everyday things feel or appear complicated, seem heavier or more difficult. It can even make our relationships with ourselves and other people feel challenging and filled with misunderstanding.

Here's an example of how this can work with physical pain: A veteran who has chronic low back pain used to enjoy going on walks with their dog. Occasionally while taking these walks, their pain has increased. Now they don't want to go on walks. They're also starting to resent the dog. Their brain has made an association between walking and pain, which turns into a generalized thought such as *I don't like going for walks* or even *Ugh, my dog is so annoying with how much work they require, and I can't handle them.*

The veteran doesn't actually dislike walks or their dog—they actually love and enjoy these things. What they *don't* like is being in pain. The pain associated with walking has become a lens through which the person sees their dog as a source of pain and irritation. Sometimes we are able to notice when this is happening in ourselves, and sometimes we need someone else's help to see it.

If you keep wearing tinted glasses, pretty soon you'll stop noticing that what you're seeing is filtered. Blue will just become part of how you see everything. Our experiences of ongoing physical, emotional, or social pain work the same way. Although the pain is filtering our experience, it can start to feel normal or like the way we've always been.

It doesn't have to be like this, however. It's possible to take off the pain glasses. You can do this by starting to be more aware of how your pain is affecting how you may be seeing and interacting with the people and situations around you. Building this kind of awareness takes practice and involves paying attention.

Here's an example of how this works. Imagine you are shopping for a new truck. You have a specific one in mind. You then start to notice that same truck when you drive around your neighborhood or park in the lot at your work. By choosing to look for a new vehicle, you've alerted your mind to pay attention in a new and specific way. Bringing attention to something helps bring more awareness. Now you're finding that truck you want everywhere.

In this book, you're "shopping" for a new perspective on pain. As you learn more about the various forms it takes, and explore your own experiences with physical, emotional, and social pain, your awareness of these things will increase. You'll be more able to see how your "pain glasses" affect your life.

You can also do this intentionally by reflecting on your pain experiences, applying this book's insights to a specific part of your life, or setting goals for increasing your awareness of your pain. The Checkpoint questions in this book are intended to help you do these things as well.

CHECKPOINT:
- What parts of your life do you see differently because of your pain?
- Who in your life might be able to help you take off your "pain glasses"?

Trauma Complicates the Mission

———

Veterans may have experienced a host of traumatic experiences through their roles and responsibilities during their service in the armed forces. In addition, their life experiences, including what happened to them before and after their time in the military, may have exposed them to trauma. This can complicate a veteran's relationship to pain and limit their ability to use healthy coping gear.

So, what exactly is trauma? Trauma is when we experience an event that either is or feels like a threat to our lives. Other types of trauma could be experiences such as sexual abuse, emotional abuse, neglect, or exploitation. We argue that trauma also includes actual or threatened loss of identity, a social group or relationship, spirituality, or anything that has emotional or psychological meaning and value for a person or group.

Trauma, like all forms of pain, is personal, cultural, subjective, and unique to each person. Trauma adds another filter to the pain lenses we just explored. It includes the physical damage and shock that come with injuries, but also emotional, psychological, and vicarious trauma that can accompany experiences of being around other people who are suffering or experiencing abuse.

Mental health practitioners and others continue to develop treatments for the effects of trauma, including PTSD. We'll discuss trauma more in later chapters as it relates to this book's main areas of focus. For now, know that while all trauma involves some type of pain, not every experience of pain is linked to trauma.

Defense Mechanisms and Disordered Coping

———

Learning about how pain works and finding ways to describe it is one thing. Making it go away is a more urgent project for most people who deal with chronic or recurring pain. As we mentioned earlier, there are healthy and unhealthy ways to do this. We'll begin by looking at some of the most common unhealthy ones. In our practice, we describe the various strategies or tricks that people develop to avoid dealing directly with internal struggles or pain as defense mechanisms.

Defense mechanisms are different from the healthy coping strategies this book offers. Positive pain management approaches focus on reducing or eliminating pain or finding ways to make living with it more manageable and sustainable. Defense mechanisms are behaviors that deny the reality of pain and struggle. When we use defense mechanisms, we're ignoring or avoiding our discomfort in the short term in hopes that it will just go away permanently. This never works.

If healthy and effective coping strategies are like precision gear, defense mechanisms are more like a cheap multi-tool. You might have a multi-tool in your pocket right now. They're okay for tightening a screw or scraping some paint off a nail head. You may even be able to hack together a small job with a multi-tool, but if you want to build a house or fix an engine, you're going to need tools more suited to the task.

As we'll explore in later chapters, some of us got our multi-tools from the military culture that shaped us or we got them from the way we were brought up as kids. Alcohol is a multi-tool. Drugs are a multi-tool. Anger and denial are multi-tools. Each of these tools may be able to address a problem at a superficial level, but they won't be able to fix the underlying issue, and you certainly won't be able to build anything new by using them.

The point we're trying to make here is that your defensive pain-coping tools may have initially helped you get through a tough situation or even a painful era of your life. But in order to take on the long-term project of building a healthier and happier life—a life that isn't controlled by physical, emotional, or social pain or compromised by addiction—you need some new and better tools.

We've identified five primary ways veterans use defense mechanisms to help them keep from dealing with pain. They include numbing, forgetting, stuffing, releasing, and displacement. While people use these disordered coping mechanisms to avoid or escape painful experiences, each actually produces unintended negative consequences that outweigh their benefit or any seemingly positive effects in the moment.

Numbing

When people experience any kind of pain, most simply want it to stop. They want the pain to go away, and if it can't go away forever, they want to not feel it. They want to not cry. To not hurt. The logic at the core of this impulse is that it's better to feel nothing at all than to feel so much pain.

It is normal to want this. Negative feelings suck. Pain sucks. But numbing doesn't just target pain and negative feelings. It can numb other emotions as well—even positive ones such as happiness, joy, excitement, pleasure, or love toward others. This is the downside to this approach. Yes, you effectively numbed your pain, but what else went numb and for how long? You likely also numbed many other feelings and parts of yourself that make you who you are.

Drinking alcohol and using opioids are two of the most common ways veterans use to numb their pain. Beyond their effectiveness at diminishing positive as well as negative feelings, these strategies come with additional health and safety risks and can drastically affect both the quality and length of your life.

Forgetting

For many veterans, the option of ignoring the past or forgetting the traumatic or painful parts of their experience in the military seems attractive. The lure of forgetting can cause you to pull out the multi-tool of alcohol or other drugs. This is especially true when something happens that sparks a memory or if you flash back to a painful event, experience, or image.

Along with forgetting comes ignoring. If you feel the need to appear strong or stoic around others, ignoring or pretending to forget your pain so others won't see your struggles can be an attractive idea. As we noted with numbing, when you use substances or addictive behaviors to forget the bad parts of your experiences, you also run the risk of cutting yourself off from good memories and positive aspects of your history.

Stuffing

We like to think of this as the whack-a-mole approach to avoiding pain. Whack-a-mole is that great carnival or fair game where you exert crazy energy with a mallet to knock various objects back into their holes as they keep popping up. The more "moles" you hit, the higher your score. When we use an addictive substance or process in this way, to stuff things like pain or fear or struggle back into their hole, we run the risk of them popping up elsewhere.

Unlike ignoring or forgetting, stuffing pain acknowledges that pain is present but actively works to keep it underground or inside. This explains why some veterans feel angry for no reason, while others feel anxious without a cause they can easily point to. Many veterans use this stuffing approach because they fear their pain will become overwhelming if it is allowed to come out into the light.

Because it requires a kind of constant vigilance and ongoing expenditure of energy (just like the carnival game), stuffing away negative emotions is exhausting. Another downside is that nothing can stay stuffed forever. At some point, our bodies tell us, "Hey, we still need to get this out somehow!" You may see the pain appear as conflict in your relationships, difficulty managing your own emotions, or even a buildup of physical pain. It's simply impossible to push the pain down forever and move forward as if it's not there.

Releasing or Exploding

The opposite of stuffing is releasing. Releasing pain? Sounds good, right? Yes and no. This approach to avoiding pain sometimes gets described as the wholesome-sounding activity of "blowing off steam." It may appear in less helpful and more explosive ways as well. Some veterans become overwhelmed with emotion, break down, and then convince themselves, *I am good now.* Some direct the emotional energy of sadness or fear into powerful secondary emotions like anger and blow up, yelling or punching things. Others may try to push their pain out through intense exercise or risky sexual activity.

Releasing pent-up pain can be part of a collection of healthy coping strategies—especially when it's accompanied by peer support or talk therapy. This can even include intense emotional expression or physical exertion. However, it can be disastrous when combined with addictive substances or processes that compromise or hijack our judgment and self-control. Trying to rid ourselves of pain in this way might offer momentary relief, but it is often followed by physical pain, shame, guilt, remorse, and even legal or relationship problems.

Displacement

Related to releasing, displacement is a defense mechanism that helps us avoid acknowledging or dealing with the true source or cause of our pain by directing intense emotions or actions onto an object, person, or idea outside of ourselves. Some veterans do this by being upset with the world, upset with the government, or upset about politics. Others narrow their focus to something really specific, even if it makes little sense from the outside. One veteran recalls getting so angry at a light fixture he couldn't repair that he threw it across the room.

Like releasing, displacement offers the opportunity to express big feelings in ways that seem safer and more socially acceptable than admitting or acknowledging our physical, emotional, or social pain and developing ways to address it openly and honestly. Until we can identify and address the sources and ongoing effects of our pain directly, however, it will stick around. Focusing and directing pain-fueled emotional energy on things or people that are unrelated to the core parts of our pain might feel satisfying, but it usually just ends up confusing and alienating people close to us.

While each of these examples of disordered coping seems to offer some kind of relief, none of them get at the underlying problem—the pain—we're experiencing. Not only does our pain persist when we use these ways of coping, but we may also create other, new problems by using them.

CHECKPOINT:

- Most of us have a few defense mechanisms in our pain management gear. Were you able to recognize any of yours in the descriptions above? If so, which ones felt familiar?
- Which of your defense mechanisms would you like to get rid of or leave behind?

Healthy Coping

———

The good news is that we can learn to do things differently. Moving from avoiding pain through defense mechanisms to dealing with it more directly and effectively is a process that includes learning and experimentation. You need to find out what works for you. Throughout this book, as we explore the realities of physical, emotional, and social pain, we'll provide information as well as specific suggestions for approaching and addressing your pain with healthier coping methods. These strategies will be part of the new gear you can add to your pain management rucksack as you remove and discard the tools that no longer serve your current mission.

Two key themes that illustrate the difference between defense mechanisms and healthy coping are proactivity and openness. These fundamental aspects of effective and sustainable pain management will show up throughout this book as we discuss positive strategies—especially in the Tangible Next Steps at the end of each chapter.

Proactive Coping

When it comes to pain or other negative experiences, there are two basic types of coping: reactive and proactive. "Reactive coping" is the standard practice for 99 percent of us, and it's the logic behind those examples of defense mechanisms we just explored. Reactive coping is essentially pain defense. Because it requires the presence of some kind of pain, it only happens when we're uncomfortable. Think of reaction as the thing we do when we accidentally touch a hot surface—we pull away (and usually shout). We start to feel physical pain or an emotion like anxiety and react by trying to make it go away. We want to hurt less or feel less anxious in the moment. Reactive coping usually also seeks the shortest and easiest path to relief.

"Proactive coping" doesn't wait for the pain to get bad. It doesn't even require pain to be present at all. Instead of responding to painful moments as they happen, proactive coping anticipates these moments. Think of proactive coping as an offensive strategy. Being proactive gets us ahead of the pain. It allows us to make choices about our response before we feel distress. It can even allow us to prevent existing pain from getting worse. In the hot surface example, proactive coping means knowing that there's a potential to get burned. Armed with this information, we can put on an oven mitt, use a tool to touch the thing, or just approach the situation with little more care and skill.

With physical or emotional pain, proactive coping might mean going for a run when we are having a great day or tackling our tougher tasks at times of day when we feel rested. Proactive emotional coping might mean talking to somebody about the stress in our life when it's minimal and manageable.

Proactive coping requires a little more forethought than reactive responses. Being proactive also demands some self-knowledge. Planning for pain requires honesty about the fact that it's part of your experience. In later chapters, we'll discuss more about the importance of accepting pain as a reality and making proactive adjustments to help manage it.

Just like offensive and defensive strategies in sports or warfare, reactive and proactive coping both serve a purpose. When we're faced with an unexpected event, sometimes all we can do is react. Reactive coping can help us deal with pain flare-ups and similar emergencies. Proactive coping anticipates the possibility of pain and helps us build a foundation for a life with fewer emergencies.

Openness

Holding pain all by yourself is exhausting! Feeling unable or unwilling to share what you're feeling or experiencing drains you. As humans, we naturally want to feel connected. When we let ourselves connect with others in ways that honor and reflect the truth of our experience, we often feel a weight come off our shoulders that we didn't even know was there. This kind of connection requires the openness that comes with speaking truthfully and comprehensively about your pain.

The first person you have to be open with is yourself. Defense mechanisms like numbing, forgetting, stuffing, releasing or exploding, and displacement are all based on avoiding reality and shielding ourselves and others from what's really going on. Openness with yourself means admitting that there are parts of your experience that you want to change for the better. It means owning the truth that you are capable of feeling physical, emotional, and social pain and that these pains are having a negative impact on the way you are currently living in the world—they are preventing you from living how you want to live in the world.

Once you can be honest with yourself about your pain, you can start to share what you know and what you want with someone else. The idea of talking to another person about personal and emotional things like pain might seem like a daunting task. Many veterans believe that if they open the metaphorical floodgates and let all the emotions out, they won't be able to close them back up again. We get that.

So here is our challenge: start small. Consider talking to someone else in very limited doses at first. Begin by finding a person who cares for you. Then try getting used to talking to this person about other things in your life—everyday events and experiences. Start with easy stuff. Too many veterans wait until their breaking point to talk. They wait for crisis moments to let their pain out, but then it often comes out in a way that it is hard to unpack or that can be easily misunderstood by others. Some veterans wait until the end of their lives to get things off their chests.

So who should you talk to? Some veterans find comfort in connecting with those who may understand their experience more readily, like brothers and sisters from their own unit. Some find it easier to talk to someone who has no connection to the military community. Whomever you choose to share your pain with, expect that, through the act of talking about your pain and experience, some of what you're carrying and dealing with may begin to feel lighter. This is not to say that sharing means all your pain will be released or resolved; it won't disappear. Still, finding connection offers real relief—and that's the mission.

Don't Give Up

—

Sometimes the struggle to explain yourself feels too hard. Saying the same thing to someone over and over again can be exhausting.

You may have already experienced this with a family member, friend, or even a health care provider who's trying to help you. Some veterans get frustrated and give up trying. You may even stop before you start and just keep quiet about your pain, thinking, *They probably won't understand anyway.*

This last thought comes up pretty often for veterans. Many of us feel that others can only understand if they have been in the military themselves. We might think only a person who has shared the same MOS or deployment can ever understand how we feel or what we have experienced. As a result, we may think it's pointless to share our experience with anyone outside this circle.

Well, that's exactly the thinking that this book challenges. The point of sharing your experience with anybody, whether they're a veteran or civilian, young or old, stranger or dear friend, is that you don't have to do this alone. It's healthy to let other people in on your experience. It helps them know and understand you better. It may seem impossible right now, but you can learn to let others see and even share the pain you're carrying—even if they can't understand all of it. As you do, you will learn more about yourself. You may even notice your own experience with pain changing or healing in the process.

If you feel people in your life don't care or can't take it, find someone who is not "in" your life to talk to. Look for a therapist. Talk to animals (dogs are great listeners, by the way). Find a vet center and talk with other veterans.

We also want to acknowledge the strength and courage it takes to open up. Many of us were taught to do the opposite—to stuff it, avoid it, or believe you are weak if you show others any vulnerability. But vulnerability is a key part of effective communication and healing. Many veterans only want to talk to other veterans. Why? The answer is often "because they will understand." Understand what? Your pain? Your emotions or thoughts? Bingo! In this way, we're being vulnerable without even knowing it!

If you are a veteran who struggles to put your feelings, thoughts, or past experiences into words, we are directly speaking to you. We imagine your reason for not wanting to talk or feeling unable to talk is a personal thing. One central idea within the field of mental health is that sometimes things need to get worse before they get better. Acknowledging and feeling pain is what we go to great lengths to avoid—and yet after we do it, we might feel better.

Tangible Next Steps

——

Look at Pain from a Holistic Perspective

Pain is not just physical. This will be a concept that will be repeated throughout the book, because it's one of the most important takeaway points we talk about. Looking at pain purely from a physical perspective is shortsighted and inaccurate. Pain is multidimensional and encompasses many areas of our lives. We feel emotional pain, for example, from grief and loss, and social pain when we're excluded or rejected or missing relationships that matter. If you haven't thought about this before, try to reframe some of your other feelings or experiences by asking yourself, *How did this hurt me?* or *What did I find to be painful about this?* In the next chapters, you will read more about physical, emotional, and social pain; however, take some time right now to jot down what you feel are some pains that fit into these categories for you. You may want to keep this list and expand upon it as you go along in the book.

Stop Making Self-Fulfilling Judgments

Thinking about how we process pain is valuable. Sometimes we come to expect pain even before it happens. Pre-determining how we'll feel or think in a situation is limiting. If we think something is going to happen, it may actually be more likely to occur. Our mindset matters. Examples of self-fulfilling judgments might be when you say, "Oh, I can't do that because I know it's going to hurt" or "This isn't a good idea because then this is going to happen."

You may have had previous experiences where this was true, but that doesn't automatically mean it will happen that way again. It's kind of like if you meet a guy named Bob and he turns out to be an asshole, you don't just go on thinking all guys named Bob are assholes. While this happens more subtly with pain, it happens pretty often. Understanding how your feelings of pain and your expectations affect your lens or perception can help you avoid overgeneralizing or making assumptions that limit yourself.

Be Proactive with Your Coping

Remember when we talked about trying to stay ahead of your pain? Some ideas for this may be to preemptively explore supports that could be helpful in various situations. Think of it like meal planning. Perhaps at the beginning of the week, you plan out what meals you will have for the week or maybe you plan something simpler like the ingredients you'll need to make a certain recipe. Let's think about managing pain and addiction in the same way. How can you plan out supports that could be beneficial in certain situations before they happen? Examples may be packing disposable ice packs in your car for your physical pain, giving yourself time to process a major difficult life event or celebrating an upcoming anniversary, or preparing yourself for a social gathering that may be new to you. Preparation can help you feel in control of something that can feel very much outside of your control.

Describe What Makes a Good Listener

Take some time to think about or write down a list of attributes that might describe someone you could talk to about your pain. What qualities are most important? Your list might include attributes such as honesty, trustworthiness, or dependability. Come up with as many ways as you can to describe a person who would be supportive and with whom you would be willing to share your story.

As you build your list, ask yourself the following questions:
- What makes you comfortable enough to share honestly?
- How can you assess this in your relationships? Is it about trust? Closeness? Relatability?
- Would talking to someone who has a little distance from the military be helpful?

Begin Talking about Your Pain

Once you have a list of attributes that make a good listener, reach out to someone who has those characteristics. Ask them to meet you for a cup of coffee and then share one aspect of your experience with them. This might be a story, how you're feeling that day, or even that you've begun to read this book. You may feel most comfortable talking to another veteran. Consider how this could be a stepping-stone for opening up to others who may be close to you.

Sharing your own subjective experience with pain may help your family, friends, or health care providers better understand you and better respond to your needs.

The fact that each person experiences pain differently may seem like a given to you. Unfortunately, most people don't understand this. It's important to remember that your pain may be linked to other life experiences that make your experience unique. You should not assume that others can understand or relate to your pain simply because of the diagnosis or the type of pain you have in common. Remember whenever you're talking with a fellow veteran that, even though they may share a similar background, they have their own unique experience and story of pain.

—

CHAPTER TWO

What Makes Veteran Pain Different?

> *In the military, the culture is to not ask for help and continue to move forward. We need to work to change this, allowing for a safe place where we as vets can feel comfortable enough to drop our packs.*
>
> **—NICK, US MARINE CORPS**

THE MILITARY HAS a long and proud tradition of withstanding the toughest tasks and missions. Military personnel are trained to endure rough conditions and to be ready to face unknown dangers. Soldiers are sent to large continents, small islands, grassy fields, arid deserts, steep mountains, deep caverns, and open oceans. They're sent to accomplish missions in these settings by means of diplomacy, shows of force, and at times lethal firepower. They prepare for all this with intense training and hard exercise, supported by branch-specific cultures that value discipline, honor, strength, teamwork, and sacrifice.

During your time in the military, you likely encountered a variety of intense or extreme experiences and situations. Some of these probably came with pain, and some of that pain may still be part of your life as a veteran.

In addition to preparing you to survive painful experiences, your training and service provided you with a range of acceptable ways to understand, talk about, and deal with physical, emotional, and social pain. These habits of mind and behavior are part of the cultural gear you got from the military. They're also probably part of the toolkit you still rely on when you think about and manage painful experiences.

This chapter explores how the reality of pain is treated in military culture and how veterans often carry these assumptions into their lives when their service ends. We'll also discuss how ongoing stigma can affect your willingness to seek help for pain and how to change your mindset about asking for what you need. Finally, we'll outline a vision for a new culture of veteran pain that respects and celebrates the ways veterans care for and encourage each other.

Military Culture and Pain

Many clinicians, authors, researchers, and even other veterans have tried to define what military culture is. One major assumption that some people make is that "culture" is one thing, and it doesn't change. Culture is usually defined as any group's shared set of values, beliefs, social norms, and behaviors. The reality is that culture is constantly evolving and changing over time. In order to become a group "insider," a person gets socialized by accepting and adopting the group's norms and values and behaviors.

Whoa! Enough with the geek speak!

Basically, culture is how everyone in a specific group is expected to act or behave. Culture helps us connect to groups and form bonds of loyalty and cohesion. These are, of course, deeply important parts of military life. One example of how this shows up in the military is that members of different branches use the same word to show their pride or to acknowledge something good. Marines say, "Oorah." Service members of other branches might say, "Hoo-uhh" or "Hooyah." While the meaning behind these words is similar, each branch has its own unique take because each branch has its own distinct version of military culture.

Culture isn't limited to group behavior. It also affects how each service member and veteran perceives and deals with personal pain. As noted earlier, pain is hard to verbalize or define. How one branch treats or uses the experience of pain is likely different from another. And members of every branch probably have some basic assumptions about what counts or qualifies as a painful experience and how they are expected to deal with it in their particular culture.

So how does the reality of human pain factor into typical military culture? One theorist suggested that military culture is based on a kind of model soldier, called an "ideal type." They summarized the qualities of this type of person with the phrase "combat-warrior-masculine" (CWM).[1]

According to CWM theory, the primary function of the military is combat, so all jobs either directly or indirectly support warfighting. Combat requires fighters, of course, so the second element of CWM assumes all members of the military should have a warrior attitude. This includes resilience and perseverance, and a mindset that projects strength and power.

The third piece of CWM identifies masculinity as the platform that best supports the first two functions. In the theory, masculinity (or hypermasculinity) includes characteristics like physical strength, aggression, competitiveness, and a resistance to showing weakness or vulnerability.

The idea behind the concept of a model soldier is that each person can get molded to reflect a specific look, feel, sound, and code of life that represents and supports the military's goals. The goal of basic training is to produce a specific type of soldier who can get the job done.

Did you notice anything about pain in the combat-warrior-masculine theory? Pain is not in the vocabulary of most models of military culture. Among theorists and among the general population, experiencing and managing the normal human reality of pain seems to get left out of the qualities a member of the armed services should embody.

How come? On one hand, pain could be used as a motivator. Pushing through pain could be viewed as a litmus test to measure strength or grit. On the other hand, admitting the reality of pain could suggest weakness. If pain is present, then something went wrong, or some part of the soldier was vulnerable in the first place.

Military training and culture issued us with a set of tools—ideas, assumptions, and rules—that were intended to be useful within the military setting to help us achieve military goals. Unfortunately, just like the CWM theory of the ideal type of soldier, many of these tools and goals leave out the reality of pain, or rigidly define it as a fixable physical problem, or push it into secret corners. These ideas, assumptions, and rules about what makes a good military member are what veterans bring home with them. It's the gear we got and the gear too many of us continue to use.

There seems to be a general understanding within military and veteran communities that the topic of pain shouldn't be discussed—at least not overtly. Not talking about pain has become the accepted and expected thing to do throughout military culture. This is especially the case when the source of pain or struggle is something invisible such as depression, substance use disorder, anxiety, PTSD, or relationship issues.

When it does acknowledge pain, military culture tends to place it in the past tense, as something endured and overcome. In this way, the military places value on certain categories of pain, such as the physical pain involved in a visible injury, while denying or downplaying the importance of other pains like loss, grief, or disconnection. In many military settings, these normal human experiences get categorized as weakness.

Nobody likes to be seen as weak; veterans and service members *hate* it. In our minds, being seen as weak or vulnerable might make us a target to be taken advantage of, a target for ridicule, perhaps even a target for more pain.

This helps explain how admitting or sharing pain may feel dangerous to veterans. We've been trained to fit in, to not be seen, and we take these orders seriously. No veteran wants to be viewed as the squeaky wheel. Sharing that you have pain or problems of any sort seems to be linked to that idea. And so we stay silent about our physical, emotional, or social struggles—or at least we have in the past. Now is the time to challenge these practices and move toward sharing our stories and finding relief.

CHECKPOINT:
- What did the military teach you about pain? How have these lessons translated into civilian life?
- How do your veteran friends or family talk to you about your pain? Are they even aware of it?
- How would you like them to talk to you? What guidance can you offer them?

Stigma Keeps Us Silent

For many of us in the military, hurting from a visible wound makes a different kind of sense than suffering from an unseen condition like depression or post-traumatic stress disorder (PTSD). Within the veteran community, physical injuries or disabilities sometimes even come with a degree of honor—we recognize what the person sacrificed. Plus, physical pain is easier to explain to others. Sometimes we might have a visible injury or physical "proof" via an MRI that such pain "really exists."

It's a shame there aren't similar devices to help us better understand the emotional and social pains veterans experience. Too often, these types of pain are treated with stigma and shame instead of respect and compassion. Fortunately, there are groups and individuals trying to change that.

Over the past century, organizations such as the Department of Veterans Affairs, Veterans of Foreign Wars (VFW), American Legion, the Wounded Warrior Project, and others have worked to remove different kinds of stigma within veteran ranks.

These organizations have created programs and initiatives that have helped to normalize veteran problems such as substance use and mental health disorders. And yet stigma remains. This is not these organizations' fault. This is not the veteran's fault. Stigma about pain or mental health or substance use disorders endures for a handful of reasons, including mistaken information about the mechanics and reality of pain and addiction, outdated assumptions about masculinity and willpower, and ongoing shame. We hide these things, and we hide how they affect us. This is a cultural issue within the military and veteran communities as well as society in general. It needs to be changed.

When everyone within a group or culture hides their pain, it's impossible to see that others are experiencing the same feeling or issue you're dealing with. If you're struggling with pain in such an environment, you probably feel very isolated and alone. For example, if you are feeling anxious in a crowded room and you look around and see that no one else is visibly anxious, you might wonder, *What's wrong with me?* Soon you start to believe that something is, in fact, wrong with you.

Imagine a veteran who believed they should be stoic and strong, based on their military-taught value systems, but after returning from the service, they find themselves crying in their room at home and have no idea why. It is almost as if the old rule (value) to be stoic isn't working anymore. It's not enough. We cannot keep it in anymore. When the dust from this battle royale settles, you may find yourself exhausted and feel ashamed for breaking down in this way. The social stigma of having mental health issues or a problem with substance use makes keeping your experience a secret feel like the best idea.

Military culture feeds into the problem of stigma among veterans when it comes to these issues. Military units operate as teams, units, groups, and squads that depend on each other, often in life-or-death situations. Within these units, if one member is not "on," they run the risk of being the reason their fellow battle buddy to their left or right gets hurt. This sense of responsibility weighs heavily on each member of the military, and this burden of responsibility often comes with us into the veteran community even though we're no longer in life-or-death situations on a regular basis.

We don't want to be "the one" who didn't deal with a situation right. We don't want to be the one who developed PTSD while everyone else in the squad seems fine. We don't want to be the one who needs to drink a fifth of whisky each night to get to sleep while others just take melatonin or need nothing at all. We want to appear strong to everyone—friends, family, and military buddies alike. We don't want to be the one who comes home damaged.

But what if you knew that many veterans deal with the same issues that you do? The answer to this question is probably different for each of you. Some of you might think, *Damn, I didn't know this was normal.* Others might call bullshit. The point here is we can be our own worst enemy when we're confronted with facts that challenge or disprove our belief that we have to suffer alone. But it doesn't have to be that way. We can learn to make decisions that support ourselves in getting help. We can imagine and build a new culture of veteran pain based on honesty, sharing, and mutual support.

CHECKPOINT:
- How has stigma about pain or addiction affected you?
- Who are the people you don't want to let down?

Asking for Help (Don't Roll Your Eyes)

—

Asking for help is often a daunting task for veterans. Veterans have had unique experiences and been exposed to situations that aren't easily understood by non-veterans. They may also continue to carry and to behave according to aspects of their training, especially when it comes to reliability and self-sufficiency.

Veterans want to be seen as survivors. We want to display strength. Most of us don't even like saying the word "vulnerability." Veterans take pride in what we have accomplished. It's not too hard to see, then, how we can also develop the idea that we don't need help from others.

Trying to understand the impact of military and veteran culture on veterans' willingness to seek help led to a research study a few years ago.[2] It involved asking veterans to choose from a list of words to describe a hypothetical fellow veteran who asked for help dealing with some aspect of life after the military. These were their top ten choices:

1. Brave
2. Honorable
3. Stressed
4. Warrior
5. Frustrated
6. Hurting
7. Missing comradery
8. Exhausted
9. Courageous
10. Anxious

These results tell a story. The veterans in this study acknowledged the reality of pain by using the words *frustrated, stressed, hurting, exhausted,* and *anxious.* They also recognized a number of admirable qualities that the imagined veteran demonstrated by choosing to ask for help. They saw this person as *brave, honorable,* and *courageous.* These warriors were willing to admit and accept their hypothetical brother's or sister's emotional, physical, and social struggle *and* they continued to see their fellow veteran as a *warrior.*

Let that sink in for a second.

The group in this study was offered a number of other words and phrases for describing the veteran who sought help. They chose *not* to use words like *unstable, alcoholic, needy, old, crazy, weak, lazy, soft, less of a man,* and *fake.* And yet these are often the words and ideas we apply to ourselves when we consider asking for help—or they reflect what we imagine others will think of us if we do.

This disconnect between the admiration and respect we seem willing to offer others who admit vulnerability and the lack of respect or care we offer ourselves in the same circumstance is part of the challenge of getting veterans the support they need to manage and live with all types of pain.

Does asking for help mean you are vulnerable? Does it mean you can't handle pain and you are weak? At the risk of repeating ourselves again, we'll just say the answer out loud here: NO! Now let's break down a few ideas that may be helpful in getting your mind and heart around the brave choice to start asking for help.

Help Just Means Help

Asking for help doesn't automatically mean that you're unable to handle the situation, nor does it mean that you want someone else to solve or fix your problem. It just means you will benefit from the assistance and expertise of someone with different skills or a different mindset than you have. Asking for help is asking someone to work WITH you to resolve a specific issue at hand. It's asking an expert to train you in on some new gear that you can add to your pack.

Thinking this way can help you shift your perception. If you struggle with anxiety, for example, and you finally agree to see a therapist, you'll soon realize that they don't take away your anxiety—that's not their job (sorry to break it to you). What therapists do is give you tools and training. They work with you to help you understand your mental health, manage your pain, and develop ways to battle your anxiety that go beyond what you've been able to accomplish on your own. By developing new skills with this new gear, you're better equipped. You'll find that your anxiety is lessened and your life is becoming a little better.

Stop Assuming How Others See You

Check the facts when you ask for help. Directly ask the person you've sought out for help whether they see you as weak, less than, stupid, or whatever other bullshit baggage you've attached to seeking assistance. Most likely they will give you a resounding NO and tell you it takes guts to ask for help. On the off chance that someone says they think your request reveals weakness or some lack of character, screw them. That person probably needs to exit your life quickly. They might even be someone who is afraid of asking for help themselves.

Most often, when we check the facts against our fears or assumptions, we will be pleasantly surprised by the response. If people know you are in pain—if they know you are struggling—then they can do something with it. Some of your loved ones have likely been waiting to be asked, and they're ready to step up.

Think and Act Outside the Box

Asking for help might include reaching out via social media, going to therapy, joining a support group, engaging in religious activities, or even trying to help another person in need. Sometimes the way to start healing and growing is by helping others find solutions and get their needs met. This also helps connect you to people beyond yourself and reminds you of the many ways that you are able to make a difference and contribute to the world around you. This insight about service to others is a valuable part of military culture and also happens to be a core component of the success behind Twelve Step organizations like Alcoholics Anonymous and other peer recovery support groups. We all need help. We all need support. We all need love and have the desire to love others. We all have shit to unpack too.

CHECKPOINT:
- Who are the people you'd drop everything to help or support?
- Do you think you give yourself the same grace and acceptance as you would give another veteran in the same circumstances as you? How come?
- What would you have to overcome or change in order to share your experience with pain or reach out for help?

Toward a New Veteran Pain Culture

It was so weird when I talked to a therapist . . . they told me what I felt was normal and I thought there was no way others felt similar to me. I got the best advice I could from the therapist. He told me I am not special and unique. I was like fuck you! But I sat on it a bit and this advice helped me realize that my issues are experienced by many veterans, not just me, and made it easier for me to reach out to vets moving forward.

—ANONYMOUS, US NAVY

The first thing to know about veteran culture is that it is *not* the same as military culture. Having said that, let's dissect it. Yes, veterans learned rules, norms, patterns of thought, values, behaviors, and mannerisms from their time in the military. The difference is that these characteristics and priorities were and are specific to the culture they *used to* be a part of. When a veteran comes home, they are *no longer in the military.*

This is more obvious for some veterans than others. There are many veterans who choose not to keep the same old haircut. Some even stop swearing (I know this is hard to believe). Many veterans lose contact with the military brothers and sisters they used to see every waking hour. Some of us take more than five minutes to eat a meal!

Unsure about how to integrate back into a non-military society, many veterans experience a form of culture shock. Some reach out to fellow veterans and develop new cultures and connections based on these interactions. They learn new social norms and expectations. Some of these are connected to military values and traditions, and others aren't.

Other veterans do not reach out to anyone from their former life. They might just give a head nod when they see another vet. Both types of veterans face the same basic questions:

- *In post-military life, do I follow the rules that got established by my experience with military culture?*

- *Do I adapt those old rules into a new way of thinking and acting?*

- *Do I completely ditch every trace of military culture and start with a clean slate?*

In one way or another, you've been answering these questions every day since you got out of the service.

As a veteran, you likely continue to value various aspects of the military culture you left behind. You may have some sense of what veteran culture is like and what you want from it. You also probably have opinions about the civilian culture around you. Each culture offers a way of seeing the world and a way of seeing your past. Each culture has a set of spoken and unspoken rules about how to talk about, cope with, ignore, or acknowledge and address pain.

You get to decide which rules from the military culture still apply to your life and which ones you can let go of, recycle, or update. Even though you didn't ask for them, your experiences of pain and trauma have contributed to your strength and resiliency. What you choose to do with your resiliency is completely up to you.

Through this book, we hope to establish a new pain culture for veterans. We especially hope to help veterans understand the benefit of looking at pain from a more holistic perspective and begin to trust that sharing pain is better than continuing to slog away at the covert mission of keeping physical, emotional, and social pain stashed away and secret. You're not alone, and you can stop believing that you are.

Here's this chapter's last word about changing out the gear you've outgrown, from this book's coauthor and fellow veteran:

When I was in high school, I wore a medium shirt. In college and graduate school, I wore a medium shirt. In the military, I wore a medium shirt. When I got married, I wore a medium-size shirt. Until recently, I wore a medium-size shirt. One day my wife (the other author) tricked me. She put a medium-size tag in an extra-large shirt! It felt great! I never knew fast food could help me lose weight (kidding)! But then I got sad. At that moment, I realized I have been suffering based on a rule. A rule that I was a medium size. I imagine you have many medium-size T-shirts in your metaphorical closets. Ideas or beliefs that used to fit you. Rules that used to apply. Coping skills that used to work. The worst part is we hold on to them in the hopes that one day, just one day down the road, we can fit into that shirt again. The moral of the story is to change your shirt. Get a different size and color. Let's fit into who we are, not who we were, in order to become who we need and want to be.

—DUSTIN BROCKBERG, US ARMY

Tangible Next Steps
—

Reflect on What It Means to Have Pain

Maybe you have never stopped to think about what having pain means to you. Take some time to do this now. Ask yourself the following questions:

- Is your pain something you try to hide from friends or family because you don't want them to see you suffering? If so, where did you learn that this was necessary?
- Are you afraid others will think you can't fix or handle pain on your own? Perhaps you don't want them to worry about you. How can you show others that you can care for yourself while also still needing help and support from people in your life?
- Do you worry about oversharing your pain? Have you been in this situation before? When and how did you or the other person handle this?

Compare and Contrast Your Military and Veteran Culture

Spend some time reflecting on the differences and similarities between military and veteran culture and lifestyles. Think about the positive aspects of these cultures as well as the parts you have problems with. You may choose to do this in a journal or notebook, or you might discuss your thoughts with a trusted friend or loved one.

Some differences are important. You wouldn't want your life as a veteran to include regularly fearing for your life, for example.

Here are some questions to consider:

- What feels okay about these differences?
- What similarities are beneficial?
- How can you remind yourself about how your military experience prepared you for your success as a veteran?
- Which aspects of military life and culture are no longer serving you or the people you care about?

Rewrite Your Story

Every one of us has a story. Veterans often enjoy telling other veterans stories about their time in the service. It creates connection, understanding, and brotherhood/sisterhood. It is validating to be noticed and heard. It reminds us that who we are and how we served are important and worthwhile.

- How often do you tell your story to yourself?
- Is it the same story you share with others?

Maybe you wrote your thoughts and feelings down somewhere when you served. Perhaps you keep a journal now. Is writing a form of expression for you? Before you throw this book across the room because we're suggesting you write your feelings down, consider this: when we write about our experiences, we get to have complete control of the narrative. We can even change the story if we want to!

You may feel haunted by your story and have no interest in reliving it. Fair enough. For some, however, shifting the perspective or changing even a few words can make a huge difference. "We failed" is different from "We did the best we could"—even if the facts are the same. You survived. Changing the frames we put around our stories and the words we use to define our experience can transform the way our experiences continue to affect us. Writing, or narrative therapy, is a powerful and healing tool many veterans use to release past pain and understand their current challenges. Think about it, and give it a try!

Let Yourself Rely on Somebody

We're often wired up to assume that our battle buddies can rely on us, but we think we shouldn't need to rely on them. It's time to let things go both ways! You might look back on your time in the military and think, *Hell yeah, my buddies can rely on me. Of course, no question!* Even now, if any one of these people reached out to you for help or advice, you would very likely respond positively and with care. How come it's so hard for us to trust that this works both ways? Let yourself believe that your battle buddies can and will provide you with the same support you'd offer them. Start with a small step. Try asking one person to help you with one thing.

Join a New Team

For many of us, serving in the armed services and becoming a veteran is one of the greatest things we have ever done. We're proud of ourselves and what we endured in order to come home to family and friends. Usually, the people we love are proud of what we accomplished as well. Our experience in the military has made a huge impact on our lives, but now that we're veterans we need to assess how it continues to affect us:

- Are there ways the tools we learned in the military are keeping us from making changes in our lives?
- Does our status as veterans create an ego or a sense that we're owed something?
- Do we feel distinctly different from everyone else?
- Has our pain become a point of pride?

It may be hard to consider these ideas or admit that they're true.

One of the most common things we hear from veteran friends, family members, and clients is some version of *Others don't understand our experience as veterans.* They assume that because others don't share the veteran experience, they will also be unable to understand their pain. Too often this leads veterans to the decision to not ask for help.

Does this sound familiar?

If so, hear this clearly: Fire yourself. Fire the belief system that tells you that no one can understand your pain. Let go of the idea that your pain is only yours and that only a person who shared your exact experience could possibly relate to it or help you learn to alleviate it. Adjust the belief that you are better than other people because you can handle tons of pain.

The truth is that pain is pain. Pain is common. Pain is normal. Pain and suffering are part of the human condition, which we share with every single other person in the world. Acknowledging this reality is an opportunity for connection, not separation. Once you accept this and fire the part of yourself that wants to stay special and suffer all alone, you can pivot to a new version of yourself. Become a new version of yourself who acknowledges that others can relate to you and help you. Then start building a support system that can work for you. Create a team that will go into battle with you to accomplish your mission.

CHAPTER THREE

Physical Pain

One morning we got up at 0500 and got ready for what was to be a crappy, rainy morning. We got our rucks ready, drew our weapons, and off we went for a ten-mile march up and down these hills that felt like mountains. The worst part was the rain. We were wet all the time. I remember we stopped about halfway through the march to eat. Half of us ate while the other half guarded. While eating, I checked on my boots. They were soaked, my socks wet from the rain and bloody from blisters that had reopened from previous marches. My feet felt like they were on fire. I changed out my socks, knowing it was [only] a matter of time—that they would get wet and bloody within minutes. This was normal.

—ANONYMOUS, US MARINE CORPS

FOR SOME VETERANS, reminiscing about boot camp or basic training brings up painful memories. Others say they loved every waking minute of it. Basic training is a time when heads are shaved or hair is cut, previously learned behaviors are unlearned, new ideologies replace old ones, and a new kind of family begins to take shape. Although the experience varies across branches of service, this period of military life often involves dealing with pain and learning new ways to survive.

The ability to endure pain is a well-respected trait within military ranks. Evidence of personal and unit perseverance provides a sense of accomplishment that gets recognized and rewarded. In basic training, the military attempts to form this mentality in new soldiers by putting them in almost impossible situations to see how they react. How many of us went on ruck marches in which our drill sergeant told us within five minutes that our battle buddy had been suddenly wounded by an ambush—and now the unit has to fireman-carry them the rest of the way?

These types of exercises prepare us to handle difficult situations based in real-world military scenarios. They also send a covert but clear message: keep going, despite your urge to slow down, to process, or even to feel. Pain is seen as an obstacle to be avoided or overcome to accomplish the mission.

This chapter explores the realities of physical pain and how we learned to ignore our bleeding blisters or simply push through the pain. We'll also discuss how this way of understanding and handling pain may be effective in the short term and appropriate for certain situations but is neither long-lasting nor sustainable. In fact, applying a boot-camp approach to pain to a noncombat life can lead to unhealthy and harmful ways of treating yourself and others.

We've already begun exploring and emptying our rucksack of old coping tools. This chapter invites you to inventory the physical pain management gear you got from the military or elsewhere and decide what's worth keeping and what needs to be set aside. Along the way and at the end, we'll also share some new tools you can try out and add to your collection.

Let's Talk Pain

——

I don't think [there's] a part of my body that hasn't hurt because of training or combat. My knees hurt almost every hour of every day. My lower back is so messed up that at one point it was suggested that I do a med board for it. I have been concussed from hatches and mortars. Knocked out cold on a patrol by a hatch falling on my head catching me right below my helmet. Running stairs and my foot bent into the angle of the step, and my big toe got introduced to my shin bone. I heard the pop. I thought I dislocated my ankle. Wrong, ruptured my Achilles. They cut out ⅞ of an inch to get good tendon to sew back together. That took a year to recover; still bugs me.

—RAY, US ARMY

Physical pain is a uniquely personal experience. Just as each person's body is different, each person's pain is felt differently. Pain can even show up differently in the same person. If we asked you about your pain, you might describe it one way on one day and use different words or images on another—maybe even in two conversations on the same day. The subjective nature of our pain experiences is part of what makes pain confusing and so often difficult to explain to others or deal with personally. Added to these factors is the complicating fact that some injuries may have occurred years ago and still present as fresh pain.

Most of us have been taught to understand physical pain as an *acute,* or short-term, issue. We're better able to comprehend pain when it seems to be short-lived and can be treated or managed immediately. Thinking about pain like this means we look for quicker solutions like surgery or medication or treatment. When someone breaks an arm, they go to the doctor, receive a cast, wait six to eight weeks, and then get the cast off. All this with the expectation that the injury has been healed and the problem resolved.

You may have experienced acute pain from injuries sustained while in the military (like shrapnel to the leg) or after the military (like getting hurt from exercising or being injured on the job). These were likely treated right then and there. By "fixing" the damaged part of your body, the pain involved was also supposed to be reduced or resolved.

We often use this approach when we take medications for our pain. We look to medications as a way to eliminate pain within a short period of time. Have a headache? Take Tylenol. If the pain is worse, take an oxycodone or tramadol. These approaches understand the solution to pain from an acute perspective. Unfortunately, veterans typically have more complex and ongoing issues with pain, largely because of the significant amount and repeated nature of the strain their bodies endured while serving. Many veterans are experiencing pain that persists, sometimes for years.

It is difficult to understand how issues with pain from injuries that have supposedly been "fixed" can continue to be an ongoing problem. Understanding this requires us to make a distinction between acute pain and its longer-term cousin *chronic* pain. We refer to pain as chronic when discomfort or suffering persists for longer than the expected duration of healing.

Chronic pain is often much more difficult to treat than acute pain, as it wears on the body as well as the mind and affects almost every aspect of a person's life. Treating chronic pain involves using multiple tools to manage ongoing symptoms that persist over time. These symptoms and their severity can also change depending on our activity level, social or work setting, or other factors that fluctuate. Dealing with chronic pain on a day-to-day basis is often draining, exhausting, and frustrating.

When talking to veterans about their physical pain, we often hear things like "I have had pain every day since I left the military." Some people also normalize their ongoing back, knee, or body pain as "what most vets have." These comments suggest an understanding that being in the military automatically means having to deal with physical pain after one's service ends.

It's essential that we understand the difference between acute and chronic pain if we're going to have a chance at getting treatment for—or even talking about—what too many veterans experience every day and assume is normal. Short-lived approaches that are used for acute pain are not going to be effective over time. These interventions may just be the start of your longer journey with pain. It can be very difficult to come to terms with this, especially when it affects your interest in life or ability to do things that you once took for granted.

Understanding that chronic pain won't respond to a "one-and-done" treatment might sound like bad news, but it can also bring some hope. There are methods for ongoing pain management that can reduce your pain to a more tolerable level and help you get back to enjoying a higher quality of life. Adding these strategies to your coping toolkit can change the way you think and talk about your pain too.

Physical pain doesn't always have a solution that happens quickly. Dealing with chronic pain requires flexibility in managing your physical symptoms as well as patience and discipline. Here's the good news: you have already developed these skills—while you were in the military! Time to put them into practice for this mission. Also, if you are a veteran who experiences chronic pain, know that you're not alone. We will offer some insight and perspective on this kind of pain, as well as additional gear—some tried-and-true ways to manage and cope with chronic physical pain.

CHECKPOINT:
- Where in your body do you experience ongoing physical pain or discomfort?
- How was your physical pain first treated? Are you treating it the same way now?
- Have you considered your pain to be chronic? What would it be like to view your pain from this perspective?

What Is Pain, Actually?

———

As we mentioned in chapter 1, pain is an experience that involves our bodies, minds, and emotions as well as our social and relational connections with the people in our lives and environment. We're taking up physical pain first, in part because that's what most of us picture when we hear the word "pain" but also because our bodies are where we actually experience and process every kind of pain.

In order to help you understand how pain-relief strategies work, we want to take a little space to describe and explain the mechanics of pain in the body. To do this we're going to go "technical manual" style for a few paragraphs. We promise it's worth the time to read.

Wherever we experience pain in the body, we feel the sensations through nerves. Human beings have trillions of nerves throughout their bodies. Each one of these nerves is networked to your spinal cord, which is plugged directly into your brain.

This brain connection may be where the saying "Pain is all in your head" comes from. Unfortunately, many people with chronic pain hear this common phrase from family or friends quite often. It can also be what we perceive our doctors are telling us, or it can even be part of our internal self-questioning when we've been dealing with ongoing pain for a long period of time. The belief that pain is simply an idea or an illusion also keeps a lot of people from telling others about their physical pain.

Let's make this loud and clear: **PAIN IS NOT ALL IN YOUR HEAD!** We can say this quite confidently. From the perspective of anatomy, biology, and neuroscience, pain is quite literally *not* all in your head! We want you to fully understand how pain works so you can combat all the voices, either external or internal, that send this message to you.

Here's the process that occurs when you experience pain: Your nerves send signals from the point of injury through the spinal cord (sometimes called the "highway for pain") to the brain. Your brain receives the signal and processes the message.

This processing happens very quickly and includes your memories of pain, sorting through sensations about intensity, your expectations about certain types of pain (how bad you may think something hurts), and even how you interpret a certain pain event. These signals are then cycled back into your body through the nerve pathways where they're reprocessed into the actual pain experience and your response to it.

We need to stop thinking that our bodies are a part of a linear system where pain travels in only one direction. The pain signals that travel the routes of our nerves and spinal cord can go in both directions, helping our bodies experience, process, and respond to painful stimuli. We experience every kind of pain with multiple parts of our bodies and brains. Misunderstanding this can lead to much frustration.

We'll revisit the importance of the spinal cord superhighway a little later in this chapter and offer some ways to use the interconnected systems of our bodies to reduce and relieve pain. For now, it's enough to note that, though our brains are a major player in how we perceive and respond to it, physical pain is not all in our heads and addressing pain well involves more than just thinking differently.

Physical Pain and Trauma

When most veterans hear the word "trauma," they imagine physical trauma. They might envision someone who is wounded by gunfire, an explosion, or other potentially lethal means, or an injury that results in the loss of a limb or other major bodily damage. But these severe examples are not the only physical traumas that military members are exposed to. Less dramatic but more common traumatic situations include loss of physical functioning from injuries sustained by exercise or exertion, accidents, age, and medical conditions, among many others.

For some people, being med-boarded out of the military due to physical impairment is an experience that is physically and emotionally traumatic—especially for soldiers who may have planned to make the military a career. These physical traumas often play a pivotal role in how former members of the military understand and engage their identities as veterans, especially if they have chronic physical pain.

Trauma in the body—which can include physical, emotional, or sexual trauma—is processed in much the same way as physical pain. It also can make pain signals more difficult to manage. When someone experiences any kind of traumatic stress, their body releases hormones that alert the whole system that something is wrong. The rest of the body responds by going into what we sometimes call "survival mode." The spinal cord superhighway is centrally involved in this reaction, just as in the physical pain response described above.

The parts of the brain that respond to physical pain are some of the same areas that get activated by trauma. Both experiences light up a reactive part of our brains that provides the body with the tools it needs to try and survive—by escaping, avoiding, or neutralizing negative or threatening situations.

You may have heard the phrase "fight, flight, or freeze." This is what's happening when the body senses that its survival is under threat. You can think of this as going into "beast mode" or "crisis mode." When our mind/body decides to "fight," it will defend itself. People in this state may start physically or verbally fighting, even if this response seems to make no sense given the situation or the people around them.

"Flight" is when our bodies tell us that we need to get out of whatever situation we're currently facing. Some people in this mode literally run or hide, while others flee or retreat by escaping or withdrawing from conversations or situations that make them feel uncomfortable. If you've ever felt a sudden urge to get away from someone or something, you know how hard it can be to ignore the "flight" impulse.

Finally, "freeze" describes how some people respond to traumatic situations; they're literally unable to move their bodies. Some members of the military have described this experience in combat, when they felt paralyzed and were unable to use the skills or responses they had trained for.

These types of trauma reactions are involuntary, biological responses. This means that *we cannot control them.* A soldier cannot predict or control whether or not they'll become paralyzed by a traumatic event, run and hide, or go into a crisis mode and fight. We have worked with veterans who find this concept difficult to accept, as they reflect on both their experiences while being deployed and their lives outside the military.

Many veterans find that they respond to normal situations with trauma reactions. Some describe responding to their spouse with anger or by fighting when they feel threatened. Others fear being perceived as vulnerable so they freeze in situations where they might be asked to share their feelings about pain, or they avoid such conversations altogether.

With all the training we received, many of us wonder, *How come I responded the way I did? Why do I still do this? Why did I not do X, Y, or Z?* It's important to know that our hardwired biology as human beings takes over in traumatic situations to help us survive in that moment.

Because of the complicated nature and significant number of traumatic situations that veterans may have experienced, sometimes these involuntary reactions show up in moments when no threat is present. Our brains can develop trauma-responsive habits that are hard to shake.

Let's be careful here. It's important to understand that even though we cannot necessarily control how our bodies respond to situations once they go into "crisis" or "survival" mode, we can learn to control how we understand these reactions and how we respond to them.

When it comes to managing and reducing all types of pain, and helping our bodies stand down from habitual trauma responses, the spinal cord seems to be a key player. This is the part of the body that we want to continually try to calm down. In order to find ways to do that, we need to understand the work that our spinal cords do in helping manage pain and what tends to make that job harder or easier.

The Paper Towel Analogy

Imagine you're holding a paper towel stretched taut between your two hands. Now imagine someone is placing pennies on top the paper towel. Stretched in this way, held on both sides, the towel is able to hold quite a few pennies without breaking. Now imagine someone starts misting the paper towel with water. As the towel gets wetter and wetter, what happens? The paper towel might be able to hold the pennies for a few seconds, but after it soaks up enough water, it weakens and eventually breaks under the weight of the pennies.

This illustrates how the spinal cord handles trauma, stress, and pain. Think of the paper towel as your spinal cord. The pennies are pain messages from chronic or acute pain. The water is trauma or stress. The paper towel may be pretty good at supporting pennies when it's dry (up to a certain point at least), and it may handle being wet just fine. However, when the two conditions occur together, the paper towel may have a more difficult time enduring the combination. In the same way, when stress, trauma, and pain occur at the same time for someone, the spinal cord and the body's ability to handle the amount of stress becomes harder and harder to manage.

These stressors can also build up over time. Our bodies remember trauma and pain. Like the weight of the pennies plus the effect of the water, these stored experiences have a compound impact on the body and the mind, making our pain worse and reducing our ability to recover between flare-ups.

Understanding this gives us even more reasons why we need to learn how to engage in strategies to support the spinal cord and body. By using techniques like deep breathing and sensory awareness (see the Tangible Next Steps later in this chapter) that help us connect with ourselves in the moment, we can create the conditions that make it possible for this part of our bodies to relax and to better manage pain and trauma.

Dealing with Pain

Like all vets, we have physical pain from all the hard work we did. From carrying heavy packs and weapons, it wears your knees, back, and shoulders down. Towards the end of my enlistment, I was having issues with all listed above and my feet. I would visit docs on my way to the shop to receive cortisone shots in my feet to combat the pain. Did I mention the ringing in my ears? Better known as tinnitus, yeah, like most I have that, and it can really throw a day off if it's bad enough. Besides this, the hearing loss has made situations like work meetings or outings with friends a little more difficult. Like many vets these pains make us feel like we are getting older a little faster than our friends.

NICK, US MARINE CORPS

Knowing about how pain works in the body is one thing. Dealing with it every day and understanding how to reduce it or make it stop is another. We will share some tools throughout this chapter to try out, but first we want to make sure you understand that there are no quick fixes. Dealing with chronic pain is an ongoing issue. This is NOT a sprint, but rather a cadence march. The good news is that you don't have to do it alone. In addition to the tips and tools we offer in this book, creating a new collection of gear to manage your physical pain may also mean seeking out medical interventions, physical therapy, and other strategies that are best administered and monitored by professional practitioners. That being said, there are lots of things you can do for yourself—in fact, you've probably already got some go-to strategies.

The Coping Question

What are some ways in which you try to bring down your physical pain currently? Many veterans tell us that they avoid certain activities or engage in tasks that may not require as much from them. Some describe simply "soldiering on," which usually means pushing through their pain, trying to ignore it, or using one of those defense mechanisms we discussed in chapter 1. Some veterans use substances like opioids or alcohol to help numb their pain or keep it from getting worse.

These are all examples of coping strategies. Some of these strategies are useful for acute pain but lose their effectiveness when pain is chronic. Some work better than others, and some come with significant risks—including addiction and even death.

As we noted earlier, healthy coping strategies combine proactivity with openness. We've found that strategies that build flexibility and strength, promote relaxation, and honor and respond to your body's ways of processing and communicating pain signals are effective, sustainable, and non-addictive.

The Opioid Answer

There are some medical interventions that were once offered as short-term strategies for managing pain that many veterans have gone on to use for longer and longer durations. The most significant and troublesome of these is opioid medications. Opioids like OxyContin or Vicodin may be helpful at some points, especially when we're dealing with acute pain issues such as while recovering from surgery or for short periods of time, but our brains and bodies were not made to handle long-term opioid use.

THE DANGER OF OPIOIDS

Because opioids are highly addictive and easily misused, these medications can also be dangerous. The Centers for Disease Control and Prevention (CDC) estimated that approximately 50,000 people in the United States died from opioid-related overdoses in 2019.[1] Provisional data from the CDC's National Center for Health Statistics for 2021 indicate that number is only growing, with more than 75,000 deaths estimated by the end of April of that year.[2]

Over the past twenty years, the problems with opioids have spun out of control. There was a specific need to react and respond to its impact on the veteran community. The VA took on that challenge during the same period, with some promising results. The Opioid Safety Initiative has increased education about opioid misuse, increased access to the overdose blocking drug naloxone for veterans and pharmacists, and improved training for VA staff. These efforts have led to lower rates of opioid prescription over the last decade, including a 64 percent reduction in opioid use among VA patients and a 70 percent reduction in patients using these drugs over long periods.[3] These numbers represent a dramatic change in the way veterans who get their health care through the VA are using opioids. One of the goals now is prevention.

Whether they utilize the VA health care system or not, veterans coming out of the military must have access to alternative solutions for managing their pain and suffering. This book is part of that effort. Non-pharmacological strategies like acupuncture, chiropractic treatments, meditation, and other relaxation techniques are increasingly available. We need to start using them. The culture of veteran pain will begin to change as more and more veterans work with health care providers and supportive practitioners to learn ways to deal with their pain *without* relying on addictive medications. This change in culture will save lives. All veterans need to recognize their role in educating themselves and each other about pain and how to manage it with solutions other than opioids or other substances.

Many veterans have been prescribed opioids for both acute and chronic pain, and some feel like this is the solution. If opioid medications have been effective in reducing your pain, it's understandable why you would want to keep taking them. They might seem like the only treatment that works on your pain. However, we urge you to ask yourself if that's really true. Perhaps this is simply the quickest way you've found to alleviate pain. There are other, and healthier, options for managing chronic pain. Let's start by examining what makes pain worse and what can help us feel better.

What Makes Physical Pain Worse?

There are a ton of ways pain can become worse. What may first come to mind is overusing the part of the body that is in pain or trying to use a part of the body that you have been advised not to. However, there are many other ways pain gets worse.

Fixation or Boredom

Even though pain isn't "all in our minds," our thoughts can and do affect the intensity of our physical pain. This is especially true when we fixate on it and when we experience boredom.

Pain can become worse when we focus too much on it. If we said, "Don't think of Santa Claus's hat," what's the first thing you'd do? Most people would immediately picture the red velvet hat with a white trim and white puff ball on the end. Just putting the word "hat" next to the name "Santa Claus" makes the image appear in our imagination. The same thing happens with pain. Once we start to think about hurting, it becomes hard to stop. We tend to fixate, which can increase the pain levels in the body.

Fixation can happen more easily when we are bored. When there is not enough on our schedule, there is a lull in the day, or work is impossible because of a pain diagnosis or other disability, we may feel bored, and this can play a major role in how our chronic pain feels and how well we're able to function. Boredom can be especially difficult for veterans who are not used to the slower pace of civilian life.

One Marine Corps veteran described the experience this way: "Going from 100 mph to civilian cruising speed, everything is done at a much slower pace. When I first got out, this was hard for me because I was moving from task to task or having a very hard time relaxing—even at a family holiday where that was the goal."

The good news is that we can use our minds and thoughts to reduce pain too. Immersing ourselves in a hobby or project—especially one that requires focus—can effectively distract us from fixating on pain or constantly monitoring whether we feel worse or better. Some veterans find relief by working with puzzles or other problem-solving challenges. Woodworking, art, or mechanics can provide helpful periodic distraction from chronic pain. Even watching TV or listening to a podcast can take your mind off physical pain for a while. Understanding the importance of managing boredom and redirecting the mind to focus on things other than pain can help you make choices that reduce pain and offer relief.

Ignoring the Signals

Let's talk about pacing. This is a huge deal for veterans with chronic physical pain. Proper pacing means that someone maintains an optimal level of functioning. Too much activity runs the risk of making pain worse, but so does too little.

Our bodies are meant to move, and when we aren't physically active enough, it can have a negative impact on our pain. This is why many people with chronic pain sometimes feel worse when they wake up in the morning. In addition to the effect pain has on quality sleep, lying still for several hours can actually increase pain and discomfort. Also, the fear of pain may lead a person to opt out of certain activities they associate with pain.

Trying to figure out what's too much or too little—finding the right pacing—can be frustrating for someone with chronic pain. It can seem like a constantly moving target. One day you may feel like you've handled your pain well and increased your activity level. Maybe you spent the day with your family, which helped distract you from the pain and you ended up doing more than has been typical for you, but then the next two days you may be paying for it.

Knowing how your body communicates—what signs and symptoms tell you when you may be reaching your limit—is a valuable skill and one that takes practice. Take inventory of yourself. What happens when you start to feel your pain? Do you know what this feels like? It may help to remember the saying "Just because I am hurting may not mean I am harming." It's okay to push past the fear of engaging in activities to keep your body active. In fact, remember your body needs movement to help with pain. Keeping this in mind, it will also be important to understand when your body is sending the signal that it's tired and needs a break. Take a second right now to check in with yourself on this. Before your pain gets worse, what are your body's telltale signs that a pause needs to occur?

Get in the habit of checking in with yourself like this on a regular basis. Soon you'll have a better understanding of how your body communicates and what it needs in terms of pacing.

Personal Stress

Personal stress is another factor that can have a major impact on pain. Stress and anxiety affect our ability to manage our emotions. When veterans feel anxious or angry, they will often notice that their physical pain cranks up. If this is left unchecked, it can start a self-perpetuating cycle of increasing both physical pain and emotional pain; we just get angrier and angrier, and hurt worse and worse.

Managing stress involves developing ways to notice when it's happening and learning how to ramp down or relax. You might also start to keep track of what events and situations tend to be stressful for you. Knowing what provokes these feelings can help you be proactive with your coping. You can strategize ways to prevent stress before it happens, reduce your exposure, or be prepared with supports. If, for example, getting to your physical therapy appointments always seems to stress you out, you can ask a friend or family member to go with you, schedule them for less hectic times of day, or find a provider that's easier to access.

The impact of stress on physical discomfort highlights the importance of understanding how physical pain and emotional pain are intertwined in the body. Have you ever gotten a stomachache when you were anxious about something? This is a classic example of how emotional symptoms play out in physical ways. Every pain is connected, even when one feels more obvious or urgent than another. We can't look at pain from a single perspective.

CHECKPOINT:
- When are you most bored during the day or week? Have you noticed any increase or decrease in your pain during those times? What do you do to fight boredom?
- Which of your body's signals for being tired are you most attuned to?
- Where would you say most of your personal stress comes from? What usually works to reduce stress for you currently?

What Reduces Physical Pain?

———

Knowing some of the things that make pain worse can help us become more aware of circumstances and situations that increase pain. The more urgent question, of course, is how can we feel better?

Treating Yourself as a Whole Person

Physical pain issues are best addressed through a holistic approach. As previously discussed, a "biopsychosocial" model of treatment is an effective approach for managing pain, as it combines medical interventions with social and emotional supports.

Medical interventions can include medications, interventional procedures like injections or nerve blocks, radiofrequency, nerve ablation, or even implantable devices for pain reduction such as a spinal cord stimulator or an intrathecal pain pump. Along with these higher tech interventions, many people with chronic pain find relief with physical therapy and alternative approaches to treating pain, such as chiropractic services or acupuncture.

Medical interventions are best used with additional support from behavioral health specialists (e.g., psychologists, substance use counselors, or social workers) to address the emotional and social stressors that often come with physical pain. Behavioral health specialists also increase a person's understanding of pain and the various strategies that can help manage pain from a mind-body perspective.

Each of these strategies aims to do the same thing: disrupt the pain signals that are traveling through the spinal cord and the brain in order to reduce pain. This combined approach recognizes that pain impacts mental health, and mental health impacts pain. It can be hard to find the seam where one begins and the other ends.

Remembering the Mechanics of Pain

As we discussed earlier in this chapter, the spinal cord is that highway where pain signals travel to reach the brain. An approach to pain management from Ronald Melzack and Patrick D. Wall called "gate control theory" tells us that there are neural "gates" in the spinal cord that either open to allow pain signals to reach the brain or, conversely, close to block the signals out.[4] We can help close the gates on this highway and reduce pain by using various relaxation and coping strategies.*

If you currently have an implantable device that helps manage your chronic pain, you may already know about gate control theory. These devices work to disrupt the pain signals to the brain via an intervention in the spinal cord. Spinal cord stimulators use electrical impulses to interrupt the pain signals on their way to the brain, and intrathecal pain pumps aim to do this with medications.

Of course, just like when you block a real highway, there is always that one asshole who goes around the barriers; the same thing happens with "traffic" along the spinal cord. Pain is not typically completely gone, but rather lessened. Throughout this book and via the Tangible Next Steps, we'll offer some specific techniques that can help regulate and reduce the pain traffic in your spinal cord and help the whole system relax and recover.

Making Adjustments

Dealing with physical pain on a day-to-day basis can seem beyond difficult. In part this is because of the way it often requires you to adjust your activities and schedule. Veterans have shared with us the frustration that comes when it seems like they must change

---

*The VA has a nice worksheet on the gate control theory of pain you may want to check out: https://www.mirecc.va.gov/cih-visn2/Documents/Patient_Education_Handouts/Gate_Control_Theory_of_Pain_Version_3.pdf.

their responsibilities at work or scale back what they can do within their home or social environments because of their physical pain.

Making these types of adjustments comes easy for some veterans, but others find this kind of flexibility difficult or frustrating. As veterans, we might value the structure and discipline we received from our military training, and we don't always like change. But when a preference for structure becomes rigidity, we can get stuck in ruts that limit our options and can even increase our pain.

There is no single solution that is going to lessen pain every time and in every situation, and there are many ways to accomplish the tasks and do the things that help us enjoy our lives and be productive. Learning the pain management skill of adjustment means being open and flexible enough to change what we think and do in order to achieve our goals. We have to learn how to adjust and adapt to the various locations, people, and situations we face every day. Developing this capacity involves some strategic planning as well as being open to change and willing to experiment. Remember, being proactive is preferable to reacting in the moment.

CHECKPOINT:

- Where do you fall on the flexibility spectrum when it comes to your willingness to make adjustments in your life to manage your pain?
- How are you able to adjust and to adapt to meet your needs when things change, or if this is difficult for you, what challenges do you find with experiencing change?

Acceptance

Along with adjustment, we also like to talk about acceptance of physical pain. That sounds shitty, we know. *Who accepts pain? Shouldn't we be fighting it?* The answer is yes, and no.

In some ways, your training in the military has helped you with this pain management skill. You learned to expect that active-duty situations would require certain things from you and might result in consequences that could be difficult and long lasting. Equipped with that kind of acceptance, you were ready to enter the fight and complete the mission.

This same attitude is beyond helpful when it comes to facing ongoing physical pain. Acceptance doesn't mean giving up; it simply means embracing what is, even when that reality includes experiences or outcomes we don't like and never asked for. For people with chronic pain, acceptance may include embracing the fact that continually using certain strategies to help reduce pain will be beneficial—even if some pain remains.

Making this kind of shift in perspective breaks a barrier for many veterans. Acceptance doesn't have to be the "end of the road." It also doesn't need to come only after years of dealing with discomfort and disappointment until you finally arrive at an "aha" in which you begrudgingly accept reality. Throw those myths out the window.

Whenever you decide to let yourself accept exactly where you're at in any given moment, you may find that both your mood and your physical pain change for the better and suddenly you see options and opportunities that didn't previously seem available.

Acceptance also often pairs with adjustment. An example may help illustrate how this works in real life. Imagine that you want to go out and watch your friend complete a marathon. Acceptance means acknowledging that your pain may limit your ability to do this without support. Adjustment means putting those supports in place so you can accomplish your goal.

In this example, you pack your back brace and knee support for the outing, as well as a folding chair, because standing on hard pavement makes the pain radiate up and down your legs and you know that five hours of that would be too much. You accept that these tools will help you be more successful at managing your pain so you can support your friend who has worked so hard to run this marathon. Adjustment in this case may also mean that you don't walk your dog for an hour after dinner that night!

Accept your limits and adjust your expectations. Also, know that acceptance isn't a one-and-done. Acceptance is an ongoing process; some things are easier to accept than others. You don't always have to feel okay with everything.

Our lives are changing all the time, and physical pain has a major impact on our emotional well-being and social relationships. Some days are going to be better than others. But, through ongoing practice, we can learn the skills of adjustment and acceptance to allow ourselves to live our best lives.

Linking Physical and Emotional Pain

We'll take up the topic of emotional pain in the next chapter, including the major impacts that grief, trauma, and various kinds of loss can have on veterans. It's important to note here, however, that feelings of loss also accompany physical pain as well.

Many veterans tell stories about how they were in the best physical shape of their lives during basic training. Maybe they lost a ton of weight or developed muscles they never knew they had. They look back on pictures and think, *Damn, those were the days.*

Without a doubt, the mental and physical transformation involved in getting through basic is remarkable. Most of us see it as one of our best achievements when it comes to our personal fitness and endurance. Our bodies worked. They did what we asked them to do and most of the time more.

Those veterans who experienced injuries after basic, either in combat or elsewhere, now have bodies that don't always do what they ask them to do. They can't take part in the fitness activities they once enjoyed. They may fear keeping up with their spouse who is active in sports and exercises regularly. They worry they won't be able to play with their kids or grandkids the way they want to because of their pain. This hurts in ways that go beyond the physical.

The expectation of being physically fit was once an essential part of who you were. Now that expectation has been flipped on its head for a reason that is not your fault. There is serious sadness that comes with this. Being perceived as someone who should be able to "keep up" but just can't can be devastating. Many veterans report feeling a deep sense of loss over the physical limitations that come with pain—including a sense of lost identity.

Physical pain also has a substantial impact on mood. When your body is managing symptoms of physical pain, everything feels off. Chronic pain can leave you feeling drained of energy or sluggish. The body's physical reactions can be off-putting and worrisome.

Veterans with physical pain often experience depression, anxiety, stress, sleeping problems, and substance use issues. Expectations of how our bodies are "supposed" to feel can make us think that we're trapped. Accepting that our bodies can't do what they used to do is difficult. Here are some common questions that may occupy veterans' thoughts:

- *How did this happen to me?*
- *Why do I deserve this?*
- *When will this go away?*
- *How will this go away?*
- *What can I control?*
- *Will this ever end?*

These types of questions are hard to answer and ruminating on them often only increases our feelings of sadness, worry, and uncertainty. As we pointed out about stress earlier in this chapter, these states of mind may make the physical pain worse. It's like the chicken and the egg—hard to know what causes what. As we become more frustrated with (and fixated on) our pain, both our physical and emotional discomfort typically increase. Our mood impacts our functioning and the quality of our life. Like the pain lenses we described in chapter 1, our emotional states affect the way we view the world and how we interact with everyone around us.

This cycle of emotional and physical pain also leads many veterans toward quick fixes and forms of relief that look more like defense mechanisms than healthy coping tools. Many try to feel better through substance use. When used as coping strategies, alcohol and other drug use may be effective in the short term—we experience a short-lived "happy" sensation when we're drunk or high—but they aren't addressing the core problems. In fact, they usually end up making everything worse.

Mood changes that come with managing physical obstacles can also cause issues with motivation. When you feel unable to do the things you'd like to, or like you used to, finding the energy to go to work, to do household tasks, or even to engage in relationships feels too hard. Decreased motivation can spiral, preventing you from keeping up with your day-to-day activities, including participation at work, school, or even at home. Better understanding what helps your motivation while dealing with physical pain can be quite valuable. For some, it is seeking activities that provide them with joy or value (an internal motivation), while for others it may be seeking some sort of reward (an external motivation). Motivation also may come from feeling accountable to someone or something.

Physical and Social Pain Connections

Many veterans with chronic physical pain describe how it makes it more difficult to engage in everyday activities with their families and friends. Normal activities like taking car trips or plane rides, throwing a football, or jumping on a trampoline with kids or grandkids can seem impossible. It's not that we don't want to do these things or haven't tried. Many are burdened by worry, wondering, *Will my pain let me do this?* Even something as simple as sitting through a two-hour movie can be grueling for someone with back pain that requires them to be up and about every thirty minutes or so.

Many of us are calculating the costs and benefits of every activity. We can't afford to let a minor mistake or overstep ruin the rest of our afternoon or evening. These situations feed a daily narrative, where we constantly ask ourselves, *Is this worth trying to do?*

The number of times we have heard veterans say, "I had to cancel that outing because of my pain" or "I couldn't do that because of *this*" (as they point to a leg or a back or a head) is saddening. For many veterans, physical pain has a major impact on their ability and willingness to connect with others socially. There are lots of reasons for this.

First of all, social connections often involve getting out to go see someone. This can be difficult if you have limited mobility because of physical pain. It can also be hard to predict pain levels on a given day, which makes it hard to plan for outings or meetups. If your pain levels spike on any given day, you might have to cancel your plans. This can be disappointing, and your friends and family might have a hard time understanding why, especially when chronic pain is the issue.

Those who have not experienced chronic pain themselves, or who have not taken the time to learn about it, may jump to statements such as "That still bothers you?" or "You said that last time—how is this still a thing?" This can make veterans resist opening up about their physical pain or even engaging at all. It often seems easier to just stay home or not explain the pain associated with the decision making.

For many veterans, taking part in physical activities can be a way to connect with others. Some spaces that expect and respect a good amount of physical endurance and strength include Cross-Fit, exercise boot camps, mud runs, and strength and conditioning sessions that are often hosted or owned by veterans. These spaces can be a natural place for veterans to meet and connect with other veterans. When someone is experiencing pain that limits their physical ability, however, the likelihood of connecting in this way may be minimal.

Often, places like bars or events like unit reunions provide accessible space to gather with like-minded friends, but those settings also usually involve drinking. For veterans who are experiencing chronic pain and also trying to manage it without alcohol or other substances, these options can be less desirable. Finding spaces for veterans to connect and socialize that take into consideration the need for accessibility and safety when it comes to substances is an ongoing challenge, but it's a challenge that can be met.

It's possible to build a healthy social network and find activities to enjoy with others, even if they require making adjustments in what you formerly did for fun. These things don't happen automatically, however. Like every other positive strategy we've shared, developing this kind of social connection requires you to be proactive and open. You have to know what you need, and ask for it or seek it out for yourself. You may also benefit from the advice and support of friends, family, and professionals.

Tangible Next Steps

Find the Right Tool for Your Pain

When you build anything, you need the right tools to complete the project. The same goes for dealing with and managing physical pain. Why use a hammer when you need a Phillips screwdriver? Finding the right tool means figuring out which pain-relieving strategies match and help reduce your pain in various situations.

For example, putting ice on a physical pain location may be effective when you're sitting still or lying down, but this is not something that's easy to do when you want to walk around or go on a hike. To do these activities, you'll need to find another tool such as a back brace or balm that provides support or relief for your pain. Perhaps sitting in a recliner is beneficial for your pain. Great! But you obviously can't take that La-Z-Boy with you to work or the grocery store.

This is where our creativity comes in. We need to gather up the many tools we have available and assess which ones fit our project—which ones work for our unique environments, scenarios, and pain types.

If your toolbox is empty or you've already tried all the gear you've got, get some help! Professionals mentioned in this chapter (i.e., physical therapists, behavioral health providers, and pain physicians or providers) are in the business of helping solve problems in a way that works for you. Your work with that person will benefit from open communication and willingness to practice new ways of addressing your physical pain.

If One Tool Doesn't Work, Try Another

We need to find the right tool for the right job. We also need to be flexible and willing to try out many tools if the first few don't work the way we hoped. Often, especially with physical pain, a single strategy may not be the magic elixir. We have to be open to the possibility that one tool may provide a certain amount of relief, but it needs to be joined in five, ten, or twenty minutes by another strategy that will help us keep managing the pain. It can be tiring to do the work required to find the mix that works for us, but it's worth it.

The longer you can keep your pain at manageable levels, the longer you can do what you want to do in your life without the pain being in control. Some examples of this multiple tool strategy might be taking medication, then lying down or trying some deep breathing, putting on music, and then icing your pain location.

Sometimes we find that people get stuck in the "acute" pain mindset (remember, this is reactive, short-lived coping) and they only try one thing. They take their medications and then get frustrated when that one tool doesn't make things better. With ongoing pain, we often need multiple tools to help reduce pain to a more manageable level.

Throw Out the Myth That Pain Is "All in Your Head"

This saying messes with so many people who have pain, especially chronic pain. We may be asking ourselves why the pain has lasted this long. Worse yet, we may have people in our lives who are saying things like "Stop being lazy" and "Get over it." We have heard many versions of this bullshit. At the end of the day these statements, and the thoughts behind them, are based on the idea that pain is made inside or only lives in your head.

If there is anything you take away from this chapter, it's that this is NOT TRUE! Knowledge is power here. Remember how pain works in the body. If you need a refresher, go back and read the "What Is Pain, Actually?" section earlier in this chapter. Pain is not an exclusively psychological or thought-based experience. There is a biological process occurring in your whole body that causes you to feel and function the way you do.

Pay Attention to What Your Body Is Saying

Just like the "check engine" light comes on in your car to alert you to a problem or potential problem, your body tries to tell you when you have become overwhelmed and need to slow down or stop or make some kind of change. Hearing, interpreting, and even more importantly listening to these messages are harder for some people than others. Many of us are used to not paying attention to these alerts; we choose to ignore them because we want to keep going. Signs and symptoms that may indicate you need to slow down come in various forms. Here are some examples:

- A physical slowing in your body. You are not doing things as fast as you were when you first started the activity. This can feel like you're losing strength.
- New symptoms that may not seem connected to your physical pain. These can include a shorter temper, emotional outbursts, crying, feeling overwhelmed, or getting in a fight with someone around you.
- Increased stress, tension, or other bodily symptoms.
- Increased use of medications and substances, which can also include alcohol and other drugs.

The next time you sense that you've pushed your limits, take some time to jot down some notes about the experience. What signs or symptoms did you notice, either during the activity or after it was over? How do you think your body tried to tell you that you should have stopped earlier?

Relax Your Mind as Well as Your Body

Many of us assume relaxation is only a physical sensation that the body experiences. We imagine lying on the beach somewhere or spending time at a lake house or cabin. Relaxation is more than that. This chapter highlighted the way the body and the mind are physically connected through the spinal cord.

We need to remember that helping the spinal cord calm down and block those pain signals requires BOTH the mind and body. Lying on a beach somewhere may seem physically relaxing, but if you're still worrying about the 10,000 things you need to do later that week or how much work you are missing, your mind is not in a state of relaxation.

Seek out activities and settings that provide rest for both the body and mind. You will find these times of relaxation to be much more rewarding and satisfying, and much more effective in reducing your physical pain. We offer two ready-to-use relaxation strategies below.

Relax by Using All Your Senses

Smell. Touch. Taste. Hear. See. Tuning in to our senses is a great way to bring our bodies back to the present and engage in a quick relaxation that doesn't have to take much time. Here's a quick tool that can help you practice paying attention to your senses.

On a piece of paper or in your mind, list the five senses. After each, write or think about things in that category that you enjoy.

Use these prompts to get started:

> **Smell:** What smells do you enjoy? What do you like the smell of in the morning, afternoon, or evening? Are there specific people you like the smell of? Are there certain places that have a distinct smell that you enjoy? Do you have a favorite scent, such as peppermint or lavender? Any food smells that make you feel good?

> **Touch:** What feels nice to touch? Is there a favorite piece of clothing that you like the feel of? What about physical touch from another person or animal? Are there certain fabrics you enjoy wearing, like silk or cotton? What supports feel good for your body? Does wearing a certain brace or compression shirt help you feel strong or more stable? Do you prefer a loose piece of clothing?

> **Taste:** What do you like the taste of? Does this change between the morning, afternoon, or evening? Do you have a favorite drink or food? Are there any nostalgic meals that you love? Are there certain flavors you enjoy, such as cherry or grape?

Hear: What sounds do you like to listen to? Are there people whose voices you prefer? What kinds of environmental sounds do you love? Are there animal noises or sounds of nature that bring you peace? What kind of music do you like? Do you have ideal music for certain situations, like when you are doing work or studying versus working out?

See: What do you enjoy looking at? Are there places you can visualize that you have been to or places you would like to go to? Do you have physical pictures you enjoy looking at—perhaps old pictures, pictures on your phone, or pictures on social media? Are there certain animals, people, or places that bring you happiness when you see them? If you were to look up a favorite place on YouTube, what would you type into the search field?

Most of us use our senses every day without much thought, but these ways of experiencing our world can also help relax us. For example, if you drink coffee every morning before work, you probably like the taste, but you may not be making the effort to intentionally notice that drinking coffee is helping to relax or soothe you.

The next time you have a cup, try taking a sip with a little added intentionality. Tell yourself, *I love this coffee and I am going to use it to help me relax.* Adding this simple step to your morning routine won't require extra time, but it may help calm your brain and ease your physical pain. These types of small intentions can make big differences in how you think and feel. This technique can work with any of your five senses.

Relax by Learning How to Breathe

We have all been told, "Take a deep breath and relax." This can be one of the most frustrating things to hear, especially when you're in the middle of dealing with something frustrating. We get it—you're already breathing.

That said, let's understand what makes a deep breath so powerful. Without getting too technical, breathing is typically an involuntary action. It's part of the body's autopilot programming. Just like the way our blood pumps in our bodies, normal breathing happens without needing to tell our bodies to do it.

However, when we *choose* to take a deep breath, we switch this involuntary action into a voluntary action. This helps turn on a built-in relaxation system in our bodies (it's called the "parasympathetic nervous system"). This powerful system interrupts and calms the fight, flight, or freeze mode we discussed earlier in this chapter.

Deep breathing is a great strategy to know about and use because it directly impacts your biology. The trick with this one is that you need to practice it and try to do it as often as you can. When you're able to catch yourself when you're in physical pain or are starting to get overwhelmed and then intentionally take a few deep breaths, it's almost always a game changer.

You'll have to practice and see how deep breathing works best for you. A general rule of thumb is to breathe in through your nose and out through your mouth. Try to breathe out for a longer amount of time than you breathe in. Some people can take one deep breath and feel a reset, while others need several deep breaths. Combining this relaxation strategy with others works well too. Try this breathing technique along with using your five senses or engaging in positive self-talk. Sometimes using a visualization with breathing can be beneficial. For example, when you breathe in, imagine smelling your favorite food or flower, and when you breathe out, imagine you are blowing out candles on a cake or blowing slowly through a pinwheel from a garden. Individuals with anxiety and pain tend to find using a visualization especially helpful, as it helps distract the mind in the moment.

Pace Yourself

Having to learn a new pace can be annoying. Most veterans got used to a certain pace while serving. We have to adapt to a very different speed of life when we come home—this is true even if we're not dealing with pain. Learning how to adjust your pace due to physical pain can make the process more frustrating and overwhelming. It can feel like trying to hit a moving target from a moving platform. Knowing this, let's expect it. Finding the right pace for you is going to be a moving target from the start.

Instead of trying to figure out exactly how long you can stand any given task or activity, try to gauge what feels consistent with where you are at that day. Maybe one day you can walk your dog for an hour, but the next day you recognize that you have already run five errands before dog walking time. Instead of yesterday's full hour, you take a ten-minute walk because you're learning to pace yourself.

As you get better at understanding and paying attention to the signs that tell you when you're reaching your limit, you can be more strategic about your pace. This can be a very effective way to manage physical pain.

Give Yourself Some Support

If you're someone who does not want to limit or strategize your pacing, then consider adding some real-life physical gear to help support your chosen activities. For example, let's say you know you're going to make an eight-hour drive tomorrow. This may not have been a big deal for you prior to your physical pain, but now it is.

You could get a back support for the seat in your car, use lidocaine patches to help with the pain, or travel with ice packs to use along the way or at rest stops. The idea here is that you can keep functioning somewhat the same as you did without pain by using supportive strategies and other accommodations to help manage your pain.

Keep in mind this doesn't necessarily mean you won't have the same pain later. Your pain may even increase from time to time, but using supports like these may help reduce your physical pain along the way and allow you to do the activities that you need to do or that are important to you.

Respect Your Limits

You may not believe you have limits. We get that. You know how it feels to be in great shape, and you're probably (and justifiably) proud of what your body has been able to do and endure. This is all true.

Let's also take a moment to enjoy a bite of humble pie here for a second. There will be times we need to swallow our pride and recognize that our pain may ask us to make one or more adjustments. If we ignore this, or refuse, we could hurt ourselves more or end up paying for it later with more or worse pain.

Sometimes we may need to say no to doing something that we want to do or choose to engage in an activity differently than we used to or how we hoped to. In addition to these practical adjustments, choosing the kind of realistic acceptance that we discussed in this chapter can be beyond helpful.

Acceptance in this context doesn't mean we love our pain and are just fine with how physical pain impacts us. This is not realistic. Acceptance here means we're choosing. We are accepting wherever we are *right now,* in the present moment. We are accepting that we need additional support or that we need to try new tools to reduce our pain to a level that feels more manageable at that moment. Acceptance goes hand in hand with validation of self. When we accept ourselves, we're validating our experiences. Acceptance means we know we're doing the best we can in this specific scenario.

Remember That Physical Pain Impacts Emotional and Social Pain, and Vice Versa

Check in with yourself every day. Consider how you may be feeling that day or what social circumstances you're dealing with. Get curious about whether these experiences are affecting your physical pain level—positively or negatively. If you notice increased stress, tension, or environmental pressures, the physical pain you are experiencing has most likely also increased.

Recognize that attacking the physical pain only from a physical perspective may not be effective when your emotional or social discomfort is also elevated. Try and tackle your emotional or social pain in that moment, which will also have a positive impact on the physical pain you are experiencing.

CHAPTER FOUR

Emotional Pain

> *After getting home, I constantly would jump up and into the bathtub for cover when I heard the big bangs from the construction equipment next door. It would take me ten to twenty seconds to realize what the fuck was happening and snap out of it.*
>
> **—CHRIS, US AIR FORCE**

> *While I was overseas, I lost several friends to enemy fire, friendly fire, and accidents. We had a situation where we lost four brothers to an IED blast. I was shocked, sad, mad, anxious, worried, and helpless. Yet, my training kicked in and I knew we still had a job to do, and I did not have time to feel. The problem was I just stayed in this mode. I never felt it was okay to let these emotions out.*
>
> **—ANONYMOUS, US ARMY**

WITHIN THE VETERAN COMMUNITY, emotional pain is a complex issue that often gets overlooked. Veterans share similar experiences of grief and loss with others in service-related fields, including law enforcement and firefighters as well as other vocations that involve risk and prioritize service. Each of these fields is based on the idea of selfless and sometimes self-sacrificial service to others.

It's honorable to live in this way. It can also reinforce the belief that you must deny yourself in order to help others. For many veterans, displaying pain or vulnerability or admitting that they need help goes against this code. They fear that expressing their feelings or admitting that they're struggling with emotional pain might add to someone else's burden, which prevents them from sharing. Your choice to hide your pain can also lead other veterans to do the same, which keeps the culture of concealment and silent suffering alive and strong.

It's time to end that. We encourage you to stop and take a good look at the emotional gear you have been carrying. Without a doubt, this gear and your training has helped you, and likely many others, survive tough times and accomplish unthinkable tasks. The gear served its purpose—but now it needs to be updated to allow you to use your strength differently.

For most of us, if we saw a fellow veteran crying or struggling, we'd likely tell them to let it out. We might also remind them they're not alone. Yet, when it comes to our own emotions, we think sharing or revealing our emotional pain won't fix our situation or that we don't need or deserve the same support for ourselves.

That's bullshit. Let's update our gear, brothers and sisters.

In this chapter, we'll shed light on the reality of emotional pain by exploring some of the emotionally charged situations that many veterans have experienced as well as aspects of military training that affect veterans' willingness and ability to express their feelings. We'll discuss some of the major sources of emotional pain for veterans, including various types of loss, and look at the ongoing effects of trauma. We'll also continue to examine the connections between emotional pain and physical pain that we introduced in the previous chapter. Along the way, we'll point out examples of unhealthy emotional coping and offer alternative tools for managing and processing this kind of pain.

It's impossible to include the full variety of emotional events and experiences that impact veterans. Each of us has a unique personal story. As you read, think about how the information in this chapter relates to your own experience with the emotional pain that comes from loss or trauma.

A colleague of ours once told us to never have tissues in our offices. At first, we did not understand her suggestion, as many patients feel emotions in our office and prefer to have tissues to wipe their tears. She responded softly by saying, "Where do those tissues go? In the trash, I assume." Then it hit us. Tissues represent what we do with our emotions. They are used to comfort yet are then thrown away. We do not want you to throw away your emotions, but rather honor the pain that comes with losing things that matter to you. In other words, let yourself feel.

CHECKPOINT:
- What do you think of when you hear the term "emotional pain"?
- What parts of your life feel stuck or unresolved?
- How do you process and release grief about the losses or trauma in your own life?

Desensitization

Emotional pain is often connected to a high-stress event or experience. This can include scary or life-threatening situations as well as sudden loss or disconnection from people or things that matter to us. From an evolutionary stance, we humans are physically programmed to recognize and reduce our emotional reactions in certain situations in order to survive.

In the military, we learn this lesson early on. In basic training, we're often exposed to stressful events, such as live-fire exercises or crisis situations. This teaches us specific reactions and operational skills. But this training is also about a process of "desensitization." Desensitization literally means "undoing sensitivity." This idea will be a key element in our discussion of emotional pain among veterans.

Desensitization comes from repeated exposure to an emotionally powerful event or experience. Over time, constant repetition normalizes the experience and makes it feel less stressful. Our bodies and minds become accustomed to these scenarios.

A common example of how this works is the way soldiers get used to hearing gunfire. The first time we hear a gunshot, most of us jump or flinch. It's normal to be startled by or afraid of loud noises, but by the time you're listening to your buddy unloading their M240 from the turret on top of your Humvee for the tenth time that day, the sound of gunfire has become normal—almost like background noise.

Desensitization is a powerful tool that helped us ignore, dismiss, and numb natural emotional and physical responses in order to focus on a mission. When soldiers become desensitized to normal human emotional pains such as fear and sadness, they may be able to function effectively and even accomplish demanding and difficult tasks, but they may also have trouble regaining or expressing these feelings once the crisis has passed.

No Time to Feel

In one of the stories that started this chapter, a veteran describes how their combat training allowed them to shut down pressing emotions including *shock, sadness, anger, anxiety,* and *helplessness* to accomplish their mission. They "did not have time to feel" in the moment. Even when this veteran did have time after the mission was over, the feelings never came out.

When we don't express our feelings in any way, they stay stuffed down. Sound familiar? There are those lovely defense mechanisms coming in again. This is the problem. In the military, we're repeatedly exposed to stressful events and emotionally demanding situations. Our training helps us do our jobs under extreme circumstances, but when the stressful event is over, many of us don't know what to do with the emotions that come up. So, often, we either do nothing at all or we stuff the event.

Again, desensitization is a useful process for making effective soldiers, but it can become the enemy as we try to face and manage the various types of pain we experience as veterans—especially emotional pain. Some people describe a feeling of being emotionally "stuck," like a light switch that has been turned off and now it doesn't work—they can't turn it back on.

One goal of this book is to help you transform the on-or-off light switch into something more like a dimmer. Rather than accepting an all-or-nothing (or simply a nothing) approach to emotional expression, we want to help you develop tools that allow you to adjust the intensity of your feelings to suit the situations you're in. This will also help spare yourself the pain and internal disconnection that comes with ignoring, suppressing, or hiding your emotions.

Loss and Grief

—

We don't like to talk about our emotions and we have a dark sense of humor. While it can be a good outlet, it can also be a cry for help.

—RUSSELL, US NAVY

For veterans, the experience of loss often leads to painful emotions that are expressed as some form of grief. Most people typically think of funerals when they hear the word "grief." We imagine or remember losing loved ones or other people (or animals) who are important to us.

We also experience grief when we lose parts of ourselves. We grieve the identities that we once had and can never get back, or past experiences that shaped us. We grieve lost connections with others. Like other types of pain, the emotional discomfort of grief is a universal human experience; however, it is a feeling that is felt differently by everyone—even if they happen to share the same loss.

It is essential to talk about grief when discussing veteran emotional pain. Many veterans continue to bear emotional pain in ways that others rarely see or fail to interpret correctly. Expressions of grief can look like almost anything, from sadness and tears to sluggishness to rage—sometimes it even comes out as laughter or jokes. Veterans often blunt the pain of grief with humor or sarcasm.

Dark humor is an important tool in many veterans' arsenal for processing painful experiences, such as grief and loss. It is often used to detach from the emotional pain that comes with remembering a traumatic experience or recalling it in conversation. For example, if veterans are joking about seeing a dead body in a street and joking about how it looked, to many people—especially civilians—that would sound awful and rude. But for some veterans, it is a way to process and to talk about something that they otherwise likely couldn't or wouldn't be able to do.

This type of humor is a defense mechanism. In the moment, it was a way to process a trauma and keep going. It was a way to survive. Underneath the jokes or the comments are feelings of sadness, fear, shock, and many other emotions. Dark humor may continue to serve as a way to change challenging emotional states into something more manageable or emotionally digestible.

Behind these outward expressions, some veterans describe feeling low or unseen and unheard. Some say they don't want to feel anything. Unwilling to display strong emotional reactions around others, they often distance themselves from grief, even though their refusal or inability to process and share their emotional pain often leads to unhealthy lifestyle choices and isolation.

Seeing this disconnection between what you feel inside and what you choose to show or share as a problem is a first step toward healing it. With practice and support, you can build a more integrated and connected emotional life that includes room for grief as well as happiness and joy. Just like with physical pain, acknowledging the reality and the impact of emotional pain allows us to start healing it.

Loss of Identity

For some veterans, joining the military was a lifelong dream. For others, it was part of a family tradition or a personal desire to give back to their country. Others joined up as an impulse decision, an emotional reaction to an event such as 9/11, or a last-ditch effort to figure out what they wanted from life.

No matter what brought them to the military, many veterans find a sense of personal purpose and meaning while serving. In the military, you belong to a specialized subset of individuals with the common goal of protecting your country. Your shared commitments help develop a bond and comradery. You become a highly functional unit in which each member has a set goal, responsibility, and job to perform. Together, you develop value systems, principles, and codes of life to live by.

In the military, you mattered to others. Your colleagues respected you and valued your contributions. You had a sense of your power, which involved self-respect and purpose and identity. Leaving a culture with such strong dynamics often creates a specific type of emotional loss. Bob's story offers an example of this.

Bob (not his real name) left the military at age thirty. He had served in the Army for twelve years and became a prominent member of his unit. He led soldiers into battle, received awards and accolades, and lost members of his squad in Iraq. He was considered one of the best leaders in his unit. One day, he learned he had a rare cancer and would be medically discharged from the military within a month. Next thing Bob knew, he was living at home with his parents and going to back-to-back-to-back medical appointments.

In many ways, Bob was fortunate. His cancer went into remission and he was able to return to the job he had before entering the Army. Yet Bob was not happy. Way back when Bob had joined the military, his friends were getting ready to go to college. By the time he got out, most of those friends had completed college, gotten married, and found careers. Some even had children or moved far away.

Although Bob worked hard in his civilian job, he had minimal responsibility, he was not in a leadership position, and his efforts were rarely recognized by others. He missed his squad and unit. He felt disconnected from his coworkers and even his family. He soon became depressed and started isolating himself.

Bob's story illuminates an important dynamic that must be considered when we think and talk about the emotional pain and even the social pain, which will be further explored in the next chapter, that veterans experience simply by leaving the military. When they return home, many veterans lose their purpose, job, support networks, and a structure that added discipline to their days. Their pre-military lives did not wait for them—things at home moved forward without them.

Although a veteran knows this logically, it can be a shock to experience and very difficult to get used to. Many do not know how to form connections in their new life. They may no longer have anything in common with their old friends. They may be single while everyone else they know seems to be married. They may find themselves looking for a new job or career while others are well established on the job front.

As veterans recognize how much they have lost in terms of shared purpose, and how different their lives have become, they feel more and more disconnected, isolated, and uncertain about their futures. Many experience this as the loss of who they are as a person. They went from living in a system of comradery, importance, and belonging in the military to an environment where these things, and the people who know and value them, are regularly misunderstood or overlooked.

Let's acknowledge that losing your identity as a soldier creates emotional pain. Although branches often suggest that the comradery and connection you feel in the military will always exist—think of slogans like "Always a Marine" or "Once a soldier, always a soldier"—the reality you face when you separate from service may feel anything but connected. Even though we still possess our identities and experiences as well as the values we embraced and the memories we created, when we leave the military, we lose our role. It's that simple. We're no longer actively contributing or being relied on. We are no longer *serving*.

Many veterans experience this as a deep-seated loss that eats at them. Some did not want to leave the military when they did. Others didn't realize what they were losing until they got home. It's important to acknowledge that going from inside to outside, from serving in the military to being a full-time veteran, can be a mixed experience at best. The emotional discomfort of this separation connects with and contributes to other forms of pain.

Processing the grief that comes from moving from soldier to veteran can be complicated by mixed feelings. There are likely a few things about your military life that you don't miss at all. Separating the parts of your experience that are worth celebrating and keeping alive from those that you're happy to let go of can be a helpful emotional exercise. Try telling someone in your life one thing about your military experience that you're happy to be done with and one thing you miss.

Loss of Spirituality

—

I remember one time we were driving down a street and heard gunfire at the end of the block. One squad tactically approached the end of the street and scanned the buildings, the alley, really anything where a person might be hiding. I looked up at a roof to my right and saw a child holding an AK-47. I had this moment of pause, as it was just a little kid. I also had to defend myself and my brothers. Thankfully, the kid never pointed it at us and dropped it off the roof. We took the weapon and entered the home, where we found a child crying with his family. When we got back to base, I started crying because I had this overwhelming feeling of how close I got to shooting a child. I always saw children as being innocent and vulnerable. My religion taught me to care for children and protect them from harm. I have two children of my own, one around the same age, and never really actually thought I would be put in that position.

—ANONYMOUS, US MARINE CORPS

When they enter the military, one of the first things soldiers receive is their dog tags. This identifier, which is to be worn at all times, lists their name, Social Security number, blood type, and religious preference. This final bit of information is used to help respect the final wishes of the soldier, should something happen to them. Dog tags are among the pieces of important physical gear that both active and retired soldiers hold dear.

Across its branches, the military community offers a wide variety of religious services to its members, respects and honors all religious practices, and continues to broaden how chaplains support all military members. Spirituality is a guidepost for many veterans while they are serving. Their religion and its practices offer a way of grounding themselves in what they know and value. Taking time out for prayer, worship, or to practice other religious rituals can offer a sense of normalcy.

When this comforting aspect of religion is threatened by events or situations that cause us to question or doubt the very basis of our faith, it can feel like losing part of who we are as a person. This is destabilizing. It can feel like we lose all control. This type of crisis can make it difficult to understand ourselves as well as what connects us to others.

What happens when a soldier is placed in a situation while serving that goes against their religion, as stamped on their dog tags? What happens if a soldier receives an order that contradicts their moral or ethical convictions? These experiences occur more often than we might realize and create a type of emotional pain that often goes unnoticed or is overlooked among veterans: the grief that comes when your faith or spirituality is shaken or seems lost as a result of your military service.

Many of us developed our spirituality through participation in the practices and community of a religion. From early childhood, many find that their religion provides meaning to life; it's also an organized way to make sense of the world. Most religions teach that killing others is bad, stealing is wrong, and being nice to your friends and family is important. Among other values, most of the world's religions seek to teach and embody love, forgiveness, humility, care for others, and respect for life.

Many people enter the military with a specific religious background and practice. Others may identify as agnostic or atheist— philosophical positions that offer beliefs and values that may not include a higher power like God.

Experiences during events such as deployment or combat can confront, challenge, or even shatter long-held belief systems. One example of this is when a soldier fires their weapon at a combatant with the intention of disarming them through lethal means. This often results in serious injury or death. Some might think, *Well, duh, that is their job,* but very few soldiers know how to feel when this situation arises and they actually have to *do* some of the things they have been prepared or trained for.

The military exposes soldiers to combat scenarios in training simulations. Some units are trained using sensors or paintballs to mimic the reality of firing a weapon at another human being. No matter how "real" these exercises get, however, soldiers know that no actual life is being taken.

The situation described by the marine at the start of this chapter—in which he was faced with the possibility of firing on an armed child—is one example of many that soldiers may experience during active duty. The drive to protect children and other vulnerable people is shared by nearly every human society, religion, and moral framework. Ongoing exposure to experiences and situations that go against this core belief can cause a person deep suffering and lead them to second-guess or question just what they believe and why. This type of emotional and psychological pain is often experienced as feelings of disgust, resentment, anger, frustration, or sadness, just to name a few.

When Value Systems Collide

A well-known example of the clash between strongly held religious convictions and military obligations in a time of war was depicted in the 2016 film *Hacksaw Ridge.* The movie is based on the true story of Desmond Doss, a soldier in an infantry unit who identified himself as a conscientious objector. Doss refused to use a weapon and take a life, as these actions did not align with his religious value system.

This young man also believed that he needed to serve his country during World War II. Basic training didn't go well for him. He was bullied by other soldiers and scorned by many of his leaders, many of whom refused to respect his beliefs. These experiences caused him emotional and physical pain. Following a judicial proceeding, it was decided that Doss could continue to serve his unit and be a conscientious objector. He was reassigned as a medic.

Doss went on to serve with distinction, saving many of his fellow comrades during heavy fighting on Okinawa even as he was wounded by a sniper's bullet. He was awarded our nation's highest military award, the Medal of Honor, for his actions.

The story of Desmond Doss sheds light on how different value systems can clash when it comes to the specific mission of the military. The soldier holds a belief, and the military holds a different belief; both are committed to the moral rightness of their perspective.

This type of clash or disconnect is fairly common, even as stories like Desmond Doss's are rare. Many soldiers push their religious beliefs down or set them aside for the collective good of their unit, the military, and their country. And we sometimes find ourselves behaving in ways that seem to go against what we once believed was true or right.

Faced with moral or spiritual crises, people sometimes redirect their painful and powerful feelings toward the original source of their belief systems, such as God or even an entire religion. We might get mad that God allowed this situation to happen. We might ask how it is possible that there can be this much death, moral injustice, or pain. We might even abandon our previous faith entirely because it fails to provide us with meaning or direction in the face of what we experienced. This can lead to a kind of spiritual crisis for many veterans when they try to reconnect with faith communities or religious practices that seem to have lost their power to comfort or guide.

After the military, many veterans might be welcomed home by family and friends who have no knowledge about the spiritual conflict and loss that their veteran went through, no idea about the actions they took to protect themselves, no idea what they saw or lost and what it cost them. Family and friends who once recognized the veteran as someone who served as a moral compass for their community or an example for others to follow may become confused about how and why their loved one has changed.

CHECKPOINT:
- What was your relationship to religion or spirituality like before you entered the military?
- In what ways did your military service affect your spirituality?
- In what ways did your spirituality or religion affect your military service?
- Is there anything you miss about your pre-military religious beliefs?

Reclaiming Spirituality

Spirituality is often seen and felt as a very personal, private matter. When our deep beliefs are rattled by our experiences or combined with grief, they can feel even harder to talk about. Many veterans struggle to share this aspect of their emotional pain with others. This is partially due to the fear of being misunderstood or judged. In many cases, it can be simply that spiritual pain is hard to describe. Others bury this type of pain deep inside themselves. Whatever the reason, spiritual pain is rarely discussed—even with other veterans. Many veterans also go to great lengths to avoid revisiting the events that led to such pain. They might try to ignore or numb these feelings through substance use or sex, while also placing blame on external entities, such as a religion. But the pain persists.

So, what do we do with this? How do we release this pain? How do we reconnect with a religion or set of beliefs that failed to protect the innocent? There's no simple answer, but there is a way to start. Find somebody to talk to. This could be a therapist, a coach, a close friend, a trustworthy family member, or a religious leader like a pastor, priest, or rabbi. Have an open conversation about how your relationship with religion has changed since you entered the military.

Faced with the prospect of having a conversation with someone about our traumatic experiences, we often fear being retriggered or even judged, dismissed, or abandoned by someone we love.

Acknowledging or admitting a past action or decision that went against our morals or religious beliefs is deeply uncomfortable. You may question whether you can or should share every detail of what happened, how it happened, where it happened, and why it happened.

If you're working with a therapist individually, you might consider and explore each of these questions. When talking with someone outside of a clinical setting, you might find it more helpful to acknowledge the loss you experienced by describing what it felt like and how it continues to make you feel. It's likely that the person across the table from you will be able to empathize and connect with you at the level of feelings and emotions, even if they cannot imagine the specific situation or events you describe. Empathy is the ability to understand and share the feelings of another. It is a huge component of emotional healing and a place to meet as one human to another. When we're met with empathy instead of judgment, we can experience the relief of knowing we're not alone and the freedom of being able to let go of some of our pain.

We often avoid these conversations out of fear. We don't want to go through the details, put words to our experiences, and admit that we're in pain. For many, these fears are all the fuel they need to stay covert with their experiences and feelings—to keep themselves from speaking about them with anyone. This always results in suffering.

As we've stated several times in this book, every human being experiences events differently, and each veteran's pain is unique. Our preexisting core beliefs, worldviews, thought patterns, assumptions, and attitudes all affect how we hold on to and process complicated emotional and spiritual pain. To process grief about religion or spirituality, you must first get clear about the importance religion or spirituality once held in your life and whether you want or need these things to be part of your life as a veteran.

If you've experienced the value of religious faith or spiritual life, chances are good that you want at least some part of this back.

You want to be able to believe in and trust something greater than yourself. You want to create meaning and have purpose for your life. Take some time to consider these questions:

- Is it fair to yourself to refuse to reconnect with spirituality based on one or more traumatic events?
- Are these events taking a connection to spirituality from you, or are you taking it from yourself because you cannot understand any deeper meaning behind your experience or justify why something happened as it did?
- How fair is it to blame yourself for events that were likely outside of your control?

These are all important questions to consider on your journey of making sense of and healing from emotional pain related to religion and spirituality.

Combat Losses

One December morning, I remember waking up early to prepare for our midday route clearance mission and noticed that the other engineer platoon had not arrived at the motor pool, as we shared the route clearance vehicles. I was called to the commander's office and was notified of a horrible tragedy the night before. The platoon had lost five men in an EFP [explosively formed penetrator] strike. . . . My platoon received the other platoon when they arrived and to this day, I can remember their faces of distraught and disbelief of what had happened. It was a somber moment/funeral and put a lot of things in perspective for me.

—JASON, US ARMY

One of the most iconic examples of grief and loss that some veterans experience comes with losing a fellow soldier in combat.

When they imagine loss in a military context, many people think of this type of event. For soldiers, this loss is profound. When you lose a fellow soldier, you lose a friend, a battle buddy, and a brother or sister. You lose someone who has gone through the same shit day in and day out, the same pain and sweat that you've experienced.

Military training prepares soldiers to work effectively as a unit to both protect each other from danger and accomplish the mission. When a fellow soldier dies, those who survived the event often suffer grief that is complicated by deep personal questions and second-guessing: *How did this happen? Why did I survive when they didn't? What could have been done differently?* These questions often turn to self-defeating statements: *It's all my fault, If only I did this,* or *I don't deserve to live when they did not.* These feelings of regret, survivor's guilt, and shame are common, and if they go unchallenged, uncorrected, and unprocessed, they can haunt a person for years. For many veterans, anniversaries of these losses are moments when grief can be especially intense.

This demonstrates what makes it so important to find ways to share and process our pain related to grief. But how are veterans expected to deal with this type of pain, when we haven't received any formal training on it? Is enduring loss and suffering grief just part of what we signed up for and we should automatically know how to do? We say no. Joining the military and making it through basic training isn't enough to prepare you for processing all the tough feelings and pain that come with losing someone in combat. You were trained in survival strategies—things like staying focused, moving forward, and stuffing down or setting aside feelings and expressions of grief—that may have helped keep you and your brothers and sisters alive during the crisis moments of combat, but those moments have passed. These approaches to dealing with the emotional pain of grief are not effective in the long term and are no longer the best ways to deal with this kind of pain.

The work you need to do now is not something you need to handle by yourself. Grief is meant to be shared. Dealing with emotional pain requires the tools of support and connection. Feeling alone in grief is isolating and often makes feelings of loss seem bigger and more profound. Connection and support may not necessarily mean talking; it's more about feeling close to others at a time when the distance between us and our lost brother or sister seems unbearable.

Anniversaries of combat losses can be opportunities for veterans to acknowledge what happened, express their pain, and connect with other veterans who share their experience. For these gatherings to be moments of healing, they need to be treated as such. In addition to looking back at what we've lost, we need to look forward toward lives that have purpose and meaning, in part because of others' sacrifices.

Loss of a Battle Buddy after the Military

As veterans transition home following military service, many try to connect with other veterans. This helps them establish a sense of comradery and connection based on a shared identity. Some veterans join social media groups or local and in-person groups such as VFW posts. Others simply stay in touch with their military friends with phone or video calls or texts.

It's usually through these networks and connections that veterans learn about what's happening in their friends' and other veterans' lives. This includes hearing about each other's triumphs, struggles, job updates, childbirth announcements, and many other life events. We often hear bad news through these grapevines as well. One of the hardest notifications a veteran can receive is that a battle buddy has died, and the worst of these is when that fellow soldier has died by suicide.

SUICIDE AMONG VETERANS

Suicide is higher in veteran communities than in the general population.[1] These statistics are well known, and often noted by the media when a veteran dies this way. Because of this dynamic, many veterans can feel misunderstood by their civilian counterparts when a fellow veteran dies by suicide. This can make veterans feel more isolated and disconnected from the non-veterans around them—precisely at a time when connection and care are most urgently needed. Remember, you are not alone and there is someone to talk to. Reach out to a fellow veteran or loved one. If you don't feel comfortable with this, call a professional who is trained in crisis care to get you through this difficult time in your life. There are many options!

If you or someone you know needs immediate help, contact the Veterans Crisis Line: call 988 or 1-800-273-TALK (8255) and choose option 1, or text 838255. Also visit www.va.gov for further resources.

News of a fellow veteran's death often arrives without warning. It can feel unexpected and difficult to comprehend. Many of us developed a sense of family and deep connection with the soldiers we served with. Veterans share strong, emotionally driven, and often traumatic experiences with one another. They learned to look after each other. To protect each other. To care and have love for each other. They also shared pain, emotions, and feelings, including sorrow, resentment, anger, frustration, disgust, laughter, happiness, and much more.

For all these reasons, whenever a veteran dies, they leave behind both a grieving family and a grieving *military* family. These sad moments often bring veterans closer together as they are reminded of the impact their brothers and sisters had on them.

Many veterans also struggle at these times, asking themselves what they could have done to prevent the death and taking some responsibility for it: *Why didn't I just reach out to her? If only I had checked in with him, then maybe he would still be alive.* This can be especially hard if there was limited contact between the veterans. In addition to the grief of losing a friend, these feelings and expressions of guilt and shame can contribute to a vicious spiral of self-recrimination that is often hard to stop.

If you're experiencing these feelings, know that another person's actions and choices are not your fault. All you can control is what you do with what you know and how you feel. Guilt and shame are often masking deeper emotions like sadness and fear. Use this opportunity to reach out to others to offer and ask for support. Doing so honors your own desire for connection and community while also honoring the person you've lost.

Trauma and Emotional Pain

Although most people think of the trauma related to physical injury whenever the word "trauma" is mentioned (see the previous chapter for a discussion of physical trauma), another significant form of trauma among veterans is related to painful emotional and psychological events. This type of trauma occurs when our sense of self—including our psyche, identity, and connection to others—is threatened or destroyed. When these emotional traumas are repeated, we often find ourselves struggling to cope or understand why or how something occurred. Sometimes this leads to self-blame, as there tends to be "no other" rational reason to explain what happened.

Witnessing the death or severe injury of another soldier is a prime example of an event that is likely to cause emotional trauma and sometimes self-blame. This is traumatic for several reasons. First, we are often watching a close friend get hurt. Second, we are usually in a very justified state of fear; the same lethal threat is near us too. Third, we find ourselves in a state of shock.

All this activates the trauma response we discussed in the physical pain chapter. In the face of such a tragedy, our brains are no longer thinking critically and creatively. Instead, they're making instantaneous, automatic decisions about whether to run (flight), fight, or freeze. There is a lot happening in a very short period of time, and as you recall, this is happening in an area of our brains that we can't directly control.

Soldiers don't have time to sit and think about what happened in the middle of a mission. We don't have time to cry or feel the pain of losing a friend. We don't have time to process, reflect, or talk through what happened. In crisis, our brains enter survival mode and then stay there, actively suppressing our human emotional processes in order to get us through the event alive. This explains why it can be so hard to describe or put words to past traumatic experiences or recall the way we felt during these events. We literally turned off the thinking and feeling machine!

Trauma can also take the form of what the mental health and medical field refers to as "vicarious trauma." Also called secondary trauma, this is trauma that comes from being continuously exposed to the traumatic experiences or stories of other people we interact with. When we have vicarious trauma, we can become desensitized to stories of trauma. It becomes "normal" to us and further shuts down our internal processing of feeling.

Within military communities, hearing about combat-related trauma is normal. It's a part of the job. Within veteran communities, sharing war stories can be healing for some, but others are further traumatized. It is important to recognize whether your environment is healing your emotional pain or further deepening it through overexposure to information or narratives that are shutting down your ability to process your feelings or connect with the person you're speaking with. Start by asking yourself how you feel in your environment. Are you anxious or angry? Do you feel numb or disconnected from yourself? Are your thoughts racing? If you can't tell whether the impact is positive or negative, reach out to someone you trust for their perspective. A counselor or therapist can also help you process your experience and put words to what you're feeling.

The unfortunate truth is that you have likely experienced some form of trauma, either as a member of the military, as a veteran, or both. This may be hard to hear. We say this not to pathologize, shame, or label you. We say this to honor your story, your experience, and your ability to persevere through tough times.

We want to acknowledge the reality that you carry underlying emotional pain. This doesn't necessarily mean you have PTSD or are haunted by your past. But it does mean that you may have experienced something that took from you, scarred you, changed you, and affected the person you are today. Many veterans know they have experienced traumatic events, but they may not be aware of how these experiences continue to impact their lives. Above all, know that it's possible to heal from trauma. Exploring the connections between your past experiences and your present thoughts, feelings, and behaviors can be part of a productive therapy relationship. Specific relaxation techniques can also help you recognize and reduce trauma responses.

It's Time for New Emotional Gear

As soldiers, we know that we need to suppress unhelpful emotions in times of high stress. We learn to remain stoic, strong, and confident—even in dangerous and difficult situations. And why? To survive. To keep our friends safe. To accomplish the mission. These behaviors are equipment we need for the job.

Veterans' gear must be different from what soldiers carry. We turn in our physical gear when we leave the military, but we might hang on to the emotional gear we used during our service. Most of us don't even know we're doing this. The reality is that many veterans don't have non-military gear that can help them deal with the ongoing emotional pain that they experience, including grief that comes with losing parts of themselves, broken or weak connections with their families and friends, and the loss of friends and fellow veterans to suicide or violence. Many veterans try to use the gear they got from military service—ideas about stoicism and emotional regulation—during times of sadness, grief, and loss. These once-useful skills are now hindering their ability to process and share emotions.

We must change our gear. We must find new gear for managing and expressing our emotional pain that fits the lives we want to live as veterans. We must learn to put down gear that is no longer helpful or necessary. Did you ever go on a mission and realize you grabbed the wrong pack, wrong gear, or more gear than was needed? We were told, "It's better to be prepared!" while internally we were like, *Fuck that—this is heavy.* You have used the same emotional gear for a long time and it served you well. Now it's time to set it down.

CHECKPOINT:
- What "emotional gear" are you hanging on to that you no longer need?
- How do you think your way of expressing emotions meets your current needs?
- What rules about expressing emotions seem to be getting in your way?

Tangible Next Steps
———

Debunk Myths about Emotions
If we're not used to experiencing our emotions, feeling them can suck. This can make us look for all kinds of ways to avoid or numb

them, including using substances, sex, or video games (to name just a few). Where did this aversion to feeling come from? Were you ever told that showing emotion is weak? Did someone tell you that showing emotion was being too dramatic? These and other myths about emotional expression seem to persist, and they can become obstacles to connecting with ourselves and others.

We often guide our behavior based on messages we have heard and the values they inform. Said another way, we too often believe myths about emotions and we fall into the thought traps that these myths create. Think hard about the assumptions you have about emotions. Figure out which are facts and which are myths that need to be debunked. Our hunch is that you are shaping your emotional life around a few myths that need a good kick in the ass.

Use the following list to start your reflection. Determine if you agree or disagree with each statement, then ask yourself what makes you agree or disagree.

- People show emotions just to get attention.
- Crying is a sign of weakness.
- When you're enjoying something, it's okay to show it.
- If you want to be respected, you have to keep a stone face.
- Being too happy just sets you up for disappointment.
- It can feel good to cry.
- Strong emotions are scary.
- Being angry is better than being sad.
- Expressing emotions is part of what makes us human.

Keep Caring

Let's say you experience strong negative emotions. For most of you, you probably say, *Fuck that* and attempt to avoid letting the emotion ruin your day. However, when you do that, you might be missing the important thing your emotion is trying to say to you. Anger, sadness, frustration, grief—they're all expressing something fundamental: you care. Emotional pain means you care, even as you want to feel better.

Feeling emotion about something—even an event or memory that is painful as hell—is a lot better than experiencing something important and having no emotion about it at all. Take pride in this! The fact that you care means you are still fighting, still trying, still living, and still have a desire to feel better. So go ahead and feel those emotions, but don't keep them to yourself! Share them with a friend, loved one, or therapist who can help lighten your load.

Give Grief the Time It Takes

In our clinical work with veterans, we have consistently heard veterans express doubt about whether they're grieving the "right way" or question why they are not "over" a friend's death or some major loss of identity (like no longer being in the military). Where do these doubts come from? Society? Our families? Our own expectations?

Wherever these ideas about the "correct" way to respond to loss came from, screw them. There is no "right way" to grieve. Give yourself some grace and be patient with the time it takes. Everyone goes through grief differently and every person works through grief on their own terms.

Imagine you're at a funeral for a friend and fifty of your closest friends and family are present. Some people are crying, others are laughing about good memories, while others are showing no emotion. Is one of these groups "doing" grief better or more effectively than the other groups? The answer is no. Everybody does grief differently.

If you feel stuck in grief or don't feel like you know how to grieve in a way that feels right for you, here are a few questions to ask yourself. We encourage you to explore your thoughts with friends, family, or a therapist.

- What do you specifically think about when you remember the person you lost?
- What emotions do you feel? What might be underneath those emotions?
- What feels unresolved for you? Did you say good-bye to this person or experience?

Honor the Fallen in a New Way

As a rule, veterans take the loss of a fellow veteran hard, regardless of who they were or how or when the event occurred. It's important to consider how we would like to honor those who have fallen, as well as our own individual and internal losses, in a way that is meaningful to us. We begin, first and foremost, by acknowledging what we lost. This may be a hard step, but once we admit or accept what has been lost, we can do something to give it respect by following a tradition based on our cultural values or religious practices, or by creating our own unique process and tradition.

All over the world, people have unique ways to honor those they have lost. Some religions have a memorial service and a burial service, and then set up a headstone to symbolize the person who passed. Many people do not believe in religion, don't follow specific traditions, or even refuse to visit tombstones. And that is okay! If you feel like the traditions you inherited aren't enough, don't seem personal, or do not fit your other losses, such as loss of self, maybe it's time to create some new traditions.

We might choose to memorialize those we have lost through symbolic means like getting tattoos, wearing veteran-related clothing, or carrying out specific traditions on the death anniversary or another significant date in the person's life. Another tradition in the veteran community is to wear memorial bracelets stamped with a fallen comrade's name and death date. Most veterans and veteran families recognize these forms of remembrance and are able to quickly identify other veterans in this way.

The process of honoring losses can be quite literal or symbolic and abstract. Here are a few other ways you might choose to honor a loss:

- Plant a tree in honor of those you lost. Visit it. Talk to it. Keep your connection with that person alive through nature.
- Wear something that represents the loss. Many veterans have bracelets they wear to identify who they lost, when they were lost, and so on. It becomes a part of who they are versus who they lost.
- Write a letter to the person or thing you lost. Be honest in this letter, and then decide what to do with that letter. Perhaps you bury it somewhere that represents the loss. Maybe you decide to burn it and give it to the air. Or you might even choose to wrap it around a rock and let it sink into a body of water.

These and other practices can feel comforting and meaningful. They can also be part of healthy grieving. But such memorialization is only part of what's involved in processing loss. Feelings of grief and pain may change over time, but they don't go away. Once you've suffered a loss like this, some degree of grief will be part of your life forever. Sometimes it gets magnified when the anniversary date approaches or arrives. Finding meaningful ways to grieve the dead can build community and help the living heal.

Reconnect with Spirituality

One major loss that many veterans experience following their time in the military is the loss of spirituality. Some are mad at their higher power for what they were put through or what they saw and how it affected or injured them. Some are mad that God would let so much pain, misery, or death occur in the world. If you suffer from addiction, for example, you may be angry or sad that a disease like addiction exists and feel like it is not fair.

On the other end of the spectrum, some veterans find that their relationship with religion or spirituality was strengthened during their time in the military. Maybe your faith was the thing that got you through the tough times. Wherever you find yourself on the spirituality spectrum, it is quite common to disconnect from religious or spiritual practices when you return home.

Here is our challenge for you: If you believe in religion, or want to believe, take a step and talk to someone about it. Maybe you start small and just talk to a friend who seems to have their spiritual practices squared away. Maybe you just walk into a religious building like a church or synagogue and take a seat to think or feel for a while. These places are often open and welcoming. Maybe you talk to a representative of the religion.

For many, finding a higher power or connecting to something that is greater than ourselves can be a powerful support in hard times. We see this in Alcoholics Anonymous (AA) and Narcotics Anonymous (NA) programs. If you're not interested in religion, that is okay too. Perhaps you'll decide that your idea of a higher power worth believing in is science or nature. The point here is to recognize that there's a spiritual part of you, however you choose to define spirituality, and then get to know it better. You might find or reconnect to a life-changing support system you never knew you could have.

Find Your People

A major issue many veterans face once they recognize that they really need to get their emotions off their chest is deciding who to talk to. Do we talk to another veteran? Should we approach a family member? High school friends? Our dog? A stranger? Whatever your answer is, be careful of pigeonholing. Do not simplify your thinking or limit your options unnecessarily.

You might believe, for example, that you can only talk to veterans about your time in the service but when you try to open up with one, they get triggered or don't want to talk about it. Then you may feel screwed! Expand your mind to include other supportive people you may have initially written off. The only way we can feel (and be) supported by others is if we let them know what we're experiencing.

If you have tried this, and the person did not care or didn't respond in a way that was helpful or respectful, screw them. Back in chapter 1, we suggested coming up with a list of what makes a person a supportive listener. Review that list now, or write one if you didn't do that exercise. Then look for a person who could be this outlet for you. Don't stop after the first roadblock; find another route. We believe in you. You may be surprised at who or what you might find to support you in your journey to end your covert mission of pain.

Enlist Professional Help

If reaching out to friends or family members to talk about the types of pain you're experiencing hasn't worked out, it may be time to find more formal help. If you feel like the problems continue or are getting worse, it's *definitely* time to enlist the support of a mental health provider. This could be a psychologist, a therapist, or a substance use counselor. If you don't know how to begin, ask your medical doctor for suggestions or referrals. They will be able to help you understand your situation and find the right kind of help.

Finding a provider can also start with your insurance or perhaps the VA system if you already use their services or are service-connected. Know that meeting with a provider doesn't mean you have to keep seeing that person. You're hiring somebody to help you. Finding a therapist or counselor you can connect with may take a few tries. You're going to feel more comfortable opening up to someone when you feel connected to them. Your provider wants the same thing. If it's not a good match after two or three sessions, no need to stick around. It's okay to "fire them" and move on. Professionals will not be offended if you decide that the relationship is not a good match.

If you believe you can only work with a mental health provider who is also a veteran, we are now speaking directly to you. It makes perfect sense that you want to work with someone who has a shared background. You'd rather not have to explain all the damn acronyms and experiences. But doesn't this position limit your options? Doesn't it include a huge risk? Not all veterans have experienced or understand combat. Not all veterans understand boot camp in the Army or Marine Corps. Not all veterans understand what it's like to stand on the deck of an aircraft carrier. Not all veterans understand chronic pain from being wounded or how much it hurts when you lose a battle buddy to suicide.

Even if our counselor or therapist is a veteran, we may very well still have to explain all our experiences. Take a second to think about that. If you have a hard and fast rule about who you're able to work with or talk to, you run the risk of eliminating the vast majority of great clinicians out there. If we were to analyze how many providers in the medical and mental health fields in this country identify as veterans, the percentage is likely pretty low. According to U.S. census data, approximately eighteen million veterans live in the United States—about 7 percent of the adult population.[2] The chances of finding the perfect veteran-affiliated provider who intuitively understands you is low.

Consider that possibly—just *possibly*—a non-veteran could help you with your health care—not because they once wore a uniform like yours, but because they understand pain, grief and loss, and addiction, and they know how to help others manage and overcome them. Most importantly, they know how to listen.

CHAPTER FIVE

Social Pain

> *When I got out, I was ready to get out. I was done with all the crap of being in the Army. I think trying to find out what to do for work was the hardest part. I tried selling cars for about six months, but I got tired of all the backstabbing that involves. It seemed like no one had any values. I used my GI Bill to go to college. I now have a good job that I am mostly happy with. I find just dealing with people is the hardest part. You cannot tell someone exactly how you feel because you could lose your job, and you have to be careful with how you talk to people.*
>
> **—MARK, US ARMY**

WHEN A SOLDIER ENTERS THE MILITARY, they are quickly introduced to an organized, oiled, and structured set of military rules, hierarchies, and expectations. Military units, whether they are active duty, national guard, or reserve, all have unit-specific cultural norms, expectations, and beliefs. Most importantly, each unit is intended to be a community that supports each member as well as the family of every soldier.

While a soldier is on a base, whether stateside or deployed, they are engaged with their military unit. They spend each day with their fellow soldiers. They eat together, have fun together, struggle together, and heal together.

Losing this structure of rules and relationships can be disorienting. Although this loss is inevitable at some point in a soldier's career, many veterans describe experiencing a period of grief after their exit from the military, even as this time often also involves feelings of joy and relief.

Most veterans return home to family and friends after their service ends. Here they begin a process of reintegrating into social settings that are often very different from the military community they left behind.

Many of us returned to workplaces, friend groups, neighborhoods, and families that don't know or value military culture and often have no idea what we experienced during our service. As we try to make sense of this, and choose how to act, and when or whether to talk about it, we may feel some discomfort and frustration others may not recognize or understand.

If you've ever been through a breakup, divorce, or even a disagreement or misunderstanding with another person, you likely have a sense of what we mean by social or relational pain. Social pain comes in many forms for veterans. We experience social pain when our hopes and expectations for ourselves or others aren't met or when we don't know where we stand or who we are in a relationship.

We experience social pain when we feel lonely or as though we don't fit into a given social setting. Social pain can be part of moving to a new home or community. It was part of the discomfort we felt during basic training when we were trying to learn and adapt to a whole new way of life.

We experience this kind of pain when we don't know or aren't able to follow the unwritten rules of a given culture, family, or group. Feeling intentionally or sometimes unintentionally exposed or excluded or shamed or bullied by a person or group is also included in the category of social pain. This pain is also connected to emotional pain, which we discussed in the previous chapter. Social pain usually leads to experiences of emotional pain and can result in symptoms like depression or anxiety.

What's distinct about social pain is that it involves relationships and connection—or lack of connection—with other people. This can include loved ones and close friends as well as total strangers. And like emotional pain, social discomfort can have a compounding and amplifying effect on all other types of pain.

This chapter highlights some of the social situations that veterans must navigate as they return home and discusses how these experiences can be confusing or difficult and even lead to conflict. Because of the many differences between military and civilian life, veterans can experience a significant amount of social pain in their everyday interactions. They seek to re-enter and re-integrate with civilian life as people who have been changed by—and are often identified by—their military service.

Many veterans have unreasonable or unmanageable expectations for themselves. They also can feel misunderstood, pigeonholed, or judged by others, which can lead to feelings of isolation and defensiveness. In addition to identifying some of the sources of social pain veterans experience, we'll explore some of the most common coping techniques—both helpful and unhelpful—veterans use to avoid or manage this kind of pain. We'll also provide Tangible Next Steps along the way and at the end of the chapter that you can use to better cope with various social pain experiences. We hope you'll use this fresh and updated gear to develop new skills in communication and connection with others that will help you get the support you need. With a little practice, you can keep social pain from limiting your life.

Comparing Social Experiences before, during, and after the Military

———

Being told when to be, where to be, how to be and what to wear is super easy. You buck up, shut up, and show up. Simple. Being in the civilian world, you have endless responsibilities and things to navigate and figure out and that can be overwhelming.

—ANONYMOUS, US ARMY

When they get out of the military, some veterans (like Mark in the example that opened this chapter) start comparing their service experience with the structure and feelings that are part of their new home, work, and social settings. The military's shared values, goals, and missions tend to build a cohesiveness and common understanding in which many things go unsaid. In civilian jobs, where ideas about shared work and responsibility aren't as strong, or don't exist at all, veterans can feel lost or adrift. Many find that their new coworkers don't share the same values and expectations about their jobs. There are real differences between doing work in which someone's life is on the line if a job is not completed thoroughly and correctly and the work done in most civilian day jobs.

In the world of work outside the military, many veterans are discouraged as they find more individualistic understandings of duty in which people mostly look out for themselves and their narrow areas of responsibility. Such realizations often remind veterans of the community they lost when they left the military and underscore the grief they feel over being separated from a unit that was guided by shared values and usually kept the greater good in mind.

Many of us also compare who we are as veterans to the people we were previously. One veteran we know, we'll call him "Bill," describes himself as "Before-the-Marines Bill," "Marine Bill," and "After-the-Marines Bill." Even though Bill left the service almost twenty years ago, he continues to explain and describe himself through the lens of his military service. Bill is proud of who he is and how he changed as a person through his identity as a marine. This is natural. Our military training and experience often include significant mental, physical, and social transformations that are worthy of respect and admiration.

Unfortunately, not all of these transformations are as positive as the ones Bill celebrates in himself. Some veterans use this before-during-and-after framework to refer to their experience of physical injury as well. You've probably heard people say things like "Prior to my head injury . . ." or "Before I injured my back I could . . . and now I'm . . ."

At best, this kind of categorization helps us understand where we stand and how we grow and change. At worst, it reminds us of what we've lost over time and what we might never get back. Even Bill's justifiable pride includes some nostalgia for the ripped, bad-ass, twenty-two-year-old he was. Whether it comes from within as we evaluate ourselves based on who we once were or is focused on how we stack up against others in similar circumstances today, comparison can become a tricky, slippery slope of disappointment and pain.

CHECKPOINT:

- In what ways is it unfair to compare twenty-two-year-old "Marine Bill" to forty-two-year-old "Veteran Bill"? How do you relate to this? What do you think needs to change?
- How does comparison work in your life? Does it help you recognize your growth as a person, or does it mostly make you angry or sad?

Managing Expectations

Regardless of which branch of service we chose, each of us who joined up had our reasons for entering the military. Maybe you have a long-standing tradition of service in your family. Maybe you were a part of a Reserve Officers' Training Corps (ROTC) program in college and wanted to continue on with a career in the military after your original service commitment. Maybe you were recruited while in high school and were the only one of your friends not interested in going to college or joining the civilian workforce right away. Maybe you decided that military service was going to be your saving grace, or was a patriotic duty, or that it would set you up with a strong foundation for life. Whatever your reason for joining, you had some kind of expectation for what being a soldier or sailor or airman or marine would be like and how it would impact or change you.

Your family or friends also had some expectations for and assumptions about what your military service would mean. In numerous conversations with veterans from every branch of service, we have found that, whatever we, our family, or our friends may have thought about how the military would affect our lives, the reality of what happened was usually quite different from what anybody expected. These differences create new dynamics that take time to adjust to.

We can't prepare for how our various experiences in the military will affect us, nor can we anticipate precisely how they will change us as individuals. What we can understand is that change is inevitable. It's also often necessary. Recognizing, accepting, and dealing with the effects of change—and finding ways to share and explore them with the people closest to you—can be a major part of lessening and healing from social pain.

Just as we had expectations as we entered the military, we also had expectations about what it would be like to be a veteran. These hopes and fears may have been shaped by our time in the service and by various perceptions (e.g., experiences of other veteran friends, stories from family, or what we have seen in the media). Many veterans leave the military with a very different understanding of their service—and of the military in general. This understanding influences what they expect to experience or receive as veterans, including recognition, understanding, support, and honor.

Some veterans come home feeling supported and respected, while others describe feeling abandoned, misunderstood, and uncared for. There's no single way that all veterans feel about anything. Our outlook on the military probably changed during our service and it may change again after our service ends. This might include how we talk about our time in the military, what we want to disclose to others about our experiences, when and how we choose to reconnect with the military community, or even how we view the wider organization.

Gaining perspective on your expectations for how you will be treated, supported, and recognized as a veteran can help you explore the reason you make certain choices in social situations. Do you get excited to share that you're a veteran? Do you feel shame? Do you feel survivor's guilt because you came home and others didn't? Is there a part of you that feels that being a veteran should be more well-respected in your community?

Understand that your expectations about the military have probably changed between the time you joined, where you are now, and even where you may be in the future. This is okay! No two veterans are alike when it comes to this perspective. It may be beneficial to explore what your identity as a veteran means to you and how you want it to matter to the people around you.

CHECKPOINT:
- What was the most important part about the military community that you lost when you left the military?

- What was the most important part about the non-military community that you gained when you left the military?
- How can you use these two questions above to help create the kind of community you want in your life now?

Your Identity as a Veteran

Being in the military came with a strong level of pride for my country and for my service to protecting our freedoms and our way of life. Finding a career that has that same feeling of extreme daily purpose is very hard. Also, the comradery is unlike any other, and very hard to replicate.

—ANONYMOUS, US ARMY

For some of us, being a veteran is just one part of our identity—one chapter in a longer story that includes other things we've done and other relationships that have shaped us. Other veterans view their experience of military service as central to who they are. How does this work for you? How does someone who steps into your life know which of your identities you hold dearest? It's easy to see with some veterans. They display their strong identity as veterans by wearing era-specific hats or shirts with skulls and flags draped down the middle. Some still wear a high and tight haircut or purchase veteran-related license plates or stickers for their cars.

While some veterans readily share their military experiences with their loved ones or social connections, others disclose nothing and avoid clothing or symbols that indicate this part of their identity. You might feel awkward or weird when asked about your military service. You might want to just move forward with your life and put your military experience in the rearview mirror. On the flip side, being a veteran may indeed be your most important identity, but others do not know this because you don't offer any cues.

If you look at your life, you likely have many identities. Some have to do with relationships (son, husband, daughter, uncle, sister). Other ways we define and describe our identities include gender, relationship status, financial status, employment status, and religious or political affiliation. Some people link their identities to the region of the country they call home or even to the sports teams they support. You likely embrace some of these identities more closely than others. Some kind of prioritization is normal and necessary. It's impossible to invest the same amount of energy into each identity all the time, and these things shift over time.

You've put more energy and focus into aspects of your identity that felt most important at specific times in your life. This includes your identity as someone who served in the military. Some of us may have made a point of identifying ourselves as veterans when we first got out of the military but are less likely to describe ourselves this way twenty or thirty or fifty years later. Whatever you feel about your identity as a veteran, it is important to consider how you will choose to communicate or share this part of who you are in your social interactions with others and how you expect them to treat you because of your service. Getting clear with yourself about how this identity continues to matter will help you communicate that to others. This can prevent many misunderstandings and disconnects that cause social pain.

The Divide between Veterans and Non-Veterans
———

Try to recall a non-military social gathering you went to shortly after exiting the military. Picture who was there, what you talked about, how you felt, and even what you were wearing. Did you feel as though you did not belong in that setting? Did you ever feel anxious? Did you often look toward the door? Did you swear a lot or make dark-humored jokes, only to find folks staring at you like you said something absurd? Did you stay silent because you didn't know what to say?

Our hunch is that you answered yes to at least one of these questions.

As we've discussed throughout this book, the military and veteran communities include specific cultural and social norms that many people in our lives may not easily understand. These may include, but are not limited to, excessive swearing, dark humor about death, and habits like regularly scanning spaces for potential threats. We're often nicely dressed, we have weird sleep habits and possess a superhuman ability to eat food extremely fast, and some of us drive so fast that it makes people afraid (you know who you are).

If these examples don't fit you, think of some social norms you learned from your time in the military that may continue to influence how you connect (or fail to connect) with non-veterans.

Many veterans are surprised at their inability to connect with non-veterans—people who don't share their experience or the cultural cues and expectations that come with military training and service. Whose fault is this? Theirs? Ours? The answer is neither—and both. Some civilians are just confused. They don't know how to interpret a veteran's behaviors. Others might make assumptions or judgments based on what they imagine about the military or what they've seen or read in various forms of media.

This is a two-way street, of course. We're also pretty good at making judgments. Our biases about civilians can lead us to say things like "If you get it, you get it" or "It's a military thing." Making dismissive judgments allows us to ignore the disconnection or deflect the awkwardness. And yet when our head hits the pillow later that night, we often feel more alone, more misunderstood by family and friends, and further isolated by these painful social interactions with others.

When we feel disconnected from others, we typically respond in one of three ways. Sometimes we double down and try harder to forge a connection; we might do this by being more friendly or boisterous or outgoing. Sometimes we back off and isolate ourselves—we avoid people and settings that trigger this feeling. A third possible response involves internalizing the issue—instead of reaching out or stepping back, we just assume there is something wrong with us.

You've likely responded in each of these ways to social disconnection in some life setting, whether in a casual social relationship, with a dating or romantic partner, at work or school, or even with other veterans from different branches, time periods, or MOS.

Bridging the divide between veterans and non-veterans requires flexibility and understanding from both sides. Your capacity to adapt and learn new skills based on new information is a powerful tool in this task. Putting this tool to work in healthy and productive ways means using some of the relaxation and pain management gear we've explored in previous chapters. Remember how important it is to be open and proactive when dealing with physical and emotional pain? The same is true with social discomfort. Resolving your relational pain will probably mean taking the first step and leading the way. You can do this.

Some People Just Don't Care—or Do They?

Serving your country is an honor for many. It is admirable and noble. It is prestigious and worthy. Yet we encounter people in the civilian world who may not believe this. Some may look at military service with contempt. In living memory, many Vietnam veterans experienced rejection or disdain when they came home. Given the national and global political unrest around that conflict, those veterans endured this dynamic more dramatically than those of us who served in more recent eras, but every generation experiences some disrespect.

Most veterans do not serve in order to be recognized or honored with accolades. We don't need or want big parades. We do, however, hope to be respected by the people in our country. Feeling like our time in the military is not approved of or appreciated by others can create a deep-seated disconnect with civilians.

In addition to those who actively disrespect our service, there are even more people who simply don't seem to care that we're veterans. Many veterans are surprised by this, and it can contribute to the social pain we experience as we try to integrate back into civilian life.

What kind of person doesn't care about veterans? The short answer is simply people who aren't paying attention. Some people don't think about the military at all. We don't need to take this personally or assume that they're doing this to piss us off.

These aren't the only people out there, though. Many civilians do recognize veterans, but they don't know how to relate to us. Some people refrain from asking you questions out of fear they will insult you or disrespect you. Still others may ask off-the-wall questions that are quite personal and totally inappropriate, such as asking whether you killed someone.

Regardless of how inept their approach may be, this interest suggests the opposite of what you worry about. Many people actually do care that you are a veteran and are grateful for your military service, but they're unsure how to show it. They don't know how to acknowledge or ask about your service in a respectful and caring way. This is not their fault, and ignorance is fixable, but miscues like these between veterans and non-veterans can be a source of social pain that leads us to feel disconnected, misunderstood, and even insulted.

These feelings are valid, of course. What we choose to do with them, specifically how we decide to act on them, is up to us. Later in this chapter, we'll offer some tips for adjusting your expectations, learning how to take things less personally, and resisting the impulse to make assumptions about what other people are thinking or feeling.

Dealing with Assumptions and Ignorance

To assume is to make an *ass* out of *you* and *me*.

You've probably heard this saying. It's a warning against prejudging situations based on what we think we know. It's an invitation to try and keep an open mind. It's worth noting that our minds usually prefer being a little more closed. Assumptions make our lives a little easier by making things seemingly more predictable. They give us a sense of what we can expect.

We could nerd out here and describe what happens in the brain when we make assumptions—how the frontal lobe tries to connect dots and discern patterns to help us feel more in control of situations and make sense of things even when we don't have all the information. This is fine when we're making assumptions about whether the sun will rise or when we want to navigate a flight of stairs without thinking too hard. This brain function works less well in relationships, however. Assuming we know what others are thinking, feeling, or going through can get us in trouble and make us miserable.

Many non-military people make assumptions about what it means to be a veteran. These assumptions often lead to misunderstandings. When most civilians are asked to name some characteristics of a soldier, for example, they usually come up with ideas that are very different from what a veteran or service member might offer.

You've likely experienced some of this, and it can be frustrating. Here are a few common examples.

"Veteran? You must have PTSD, right?"

How many times have you been typecast as someone who has post-traumatic stress disorder just because you are a veteran? What do you do in these situations? Do you kindly let the person know that not everyone who was in the military has PTSD? Do you mess with them and say, "Oh yeah, we all get PTSD—it's part of what we signed up for"? Or do you just shrug it off?

Going back into society where many assume that veterans have ongoing psychological or emotional trauma can provoke anxiety and anger. Wondering how others perceive your mental and emotional state can cause you to question your ability to engage in work, relate to your coworkers, or even meet new people.

"Your anger must be because of the military."

Hopefully by this point in the book you recognize that anger, sadness, and any other emotions do not just come from your experience in the military. Emotions are complicated; most people like easy answers. You may find yourself among people who attribute your emotions or your lack of emotional display to the military, even though there are probably more complex layers to and sources for the emotions you are experiencing.

It also may be tough to hear someone who has not been in the military blaming one of the most significant experiences in your life for your current emotions—even if it's partly true. This can feel a little like when a friend says something critical about one of your siblings—like they're annoying or too outspoken. Even if you think the criticism is true, it's only okay for *you* to say this. Many of us feel a sense of protective loyalty when someone else tries to blame something on the military, even when there may be some truth in what they say.

*"How come you still have pain? Weren't you
in the military decades ago?"*

Ah, the lovely assumption that all pain is acute and short lived. This is a double-whammy frustration. First of all, someone is assuming that you should be "over" a certain type of pain. Second, this kind of statement suggests that your military experience should not still affect your current level of functioning. This can feel like someone is ridiculing you or discounting the physical pain you endured from your time of serving.

*"Hey, you're not in the military anymore—
stop acting like that."*

All veterans accept that integrating back into civilian life will require some adjustment, but the idea that our experience is unwelcome or inappropriate isn't fair. Should a veteran have to hide their military identity to avoid being labeled as a hard-ass, or rigid, or set in their ways? Absolutely not. Some of the characteristics and qualities we gained from military training and service are quite helpful in various settings and environments outside the military. Embracing the positive and productive aspects of our identities can help veterans and civilians connect and appreciate each other's gifts and contributions.

Choosing Our Responses

So how do we receive the assumptions that others make about us because we're veterans, and what do we do with this information? Many veterans describe feeling disappointed, hurt, or angry. These can be valid initial responses, but staying in these emotions almost always leads to continued frustration, which can show up as intolerance or even rage. This only perpetuates cycles of hurt feelings and misunderstanding.

We can start by examining our own assumptions. Many veterans may also have ideas about what it means to be a civilian and make assumptions about what people know or don't know or what they value or care about. As tempting and as easy as this is, it's also immature and counterproductive. We need to stop putting ourselves and others into categories and reducing everybody to a label. No one fits perfectly in a box or completely exemplifies what it means to be anything.

One way to live this out is to treat others the way we prefer to be treated. Doing so is one way of communicating your expectations to another person while also respecting them as a unique individual.

When it comes to assumptions—yours or someone else's—ignorance is the enemy and education is power. For others to understand how you feel about what they're saying or suggesting by their actions, you need to speak up and let them in. Likewise, changing your own assumptions about others requires you to learn as well, which means asking questions and listening to answers. This can be quite powerful, even if it takes time and effort.

In cases where this kind of conversation is not possible or not likely to change anything, learning how to choose your response instead of reacting from a place of pain may help you stay out of trouble, or at least not make things worse. Even something as simple as counting to ten or excusing yourself from a conversation or situation can help you relax and recalibrate. Debriefing or processing your thoughts and feelings after the fact with a trusted friend or counselor may help you approach similar situations with a wider perspective and more options.

As we mentioned earlier, assumptions usually come from people trying to make connections and draw conclusions when they don't have all the information. When we recognize this, we can start to get a picture of what people misunderstand about veterans and service members. Other times, people may be missing information, have wrong information, or have not had the opportunity to learn about a population that is different from them. We've all done this in one form or another. This fact doesn't make it right; it just makes us human.

CHECKPOINT:
- What can you do when faced with others' ignorance about the military and veteran communities?
- What role should veterans play in helping inform people about our experience?
- How can you communicate the way you'd like to be treated by others?
- What do you still need to learn about civilian life?

Crisis and Conflict—Where the Trauma Response Shows Up

If you take a look back at your glorious time of basic training (kidding), your memories likely include the stress and pain you endured. Exercises and events such as taking on the pit, getting smoked, long nights, short sleeps, barely edible food, drinking more water than ever before, and gagging on your breath as you took off your NBC gear after leaving the gas chamber are all parts of the training that prepares soldiers to persist in difficult and dangerous situations.

We did these things so we could survive when we ran into worse kinds of trouble. Our training prepared us to persevere, to help our battle buddies, and to complete our missions. The moment-to-moment goal of survival was tattooed on our soul. It became so much a part of us that we brought it to every mission we needed to accomplish. Some of us still approach life with that same survival mentality that comes with being a soldier. But as veterans, we may find this well-intentioned approach can work against us now that the threats we trained for have been replaced by the challenges of civilian life.

Survival mentality is linked to those trauma responses we discussed in the previous chapters on physical and emotional pain. It's part of our human biology, which works to protect us and the people and things we care about. Switching into survival mode helps us avoid or overcome danger so we can keep on living.

Our human impulse to survive stops helping and starts hurting, however, when it moves from being an occasional response necessitated by a high-stress event to a habitual response to everyday problems. When a person feels as though their survival is always at stake in every situation, they tend to view everything as a big deal. This is especially true when something goes wrong or when a relationship experiences tension or conflict.

When we live our lives in active survival mode, we feel tense and on edge, even when the situation doesn't call for these feelings. Have you ever felt like your head is on a swivel as you constantly try to anticipate threats or guard others who seem vulnerable? Our intentions are good, maybe. And yet we are not okay. Living in survival mode long term is hard on us, and it can be a disaster for relationships.

Constantly looking at all events with a prepare-for-the-worst high intensity is exhausting. It creates an unreasonable pressure for vigilance that humans cannot sustain. This can create anxiety that will be quite difficult to cope with. So, what can we do? Do we continue on this path and respond to every conflict as though it were life-threatening? Hopefully not. The goal here is to reflect on what gets to be called a "crisis" and recalibrate our responses and behaviors.

For any of you former gunners out there, it's like finding a target and then deciding which ammunition you want to use. If all situations that involve discomfort are perceived as life-or-death threats, we will put all our energy into neutralizing the threat, and we won't be able to live our life very well or with much happiness. This can also affect your loved ones' happiness. Being around somebody who functions in this way is often frightening or exhausting.

Remember, the best antidote to any kind of pain is relaxation, but there's no room to relax in survival mode. Later in this chapter we will outline some concrete ways to challenge the survival mindset and help yourself stand down.

Concealment Is a Social Strategy

I was on the phone with someone from my family while I was deployed. An IED went off in the near distance, and my family member immediately asked me, "What was that? Are you okay?" I quickly knew I needed to get off the phone without alarming my family members and without them thinking anything was wrong.

—ANONYMOUS, US AIR FORCE

Concealing our condition or our need for help from others is the most common coping strategy veterans use to manage physical, emotional, and social pain. The lack of discussion around pain has become part of veteran culture, which is rooted in military expectations about strength and endurance through adversity and training in unit cohesion. Refusing to admit or disclose anything that might be perceived as weakness or vulnerability has turned into an automatic shield of protection for too many of us.

As we've noted throughout this book, stuffing down your pain and misery or setting it aside for a future reckoning might have helped you get through basic or your time serving, and it might even be the right choice in an extreme crisis, but as a strategy for healing, reducing, or resolving pain, concealment sucks. The mission of learning to live with and manage pain and painful experiences is not meant to be a covert mission or a solo journey. We're supposed to do this together.

This leads to another big reason veterans conceal their pain: we don't want to be a burden to others. Along with our aversion to being perceived as vulnerable, most of us were trained to value the functioning of our unit above all. We were taught to fit in and serve the unit by putting others first. Being the squeaky wheel or the person our battle buddies had to carry or accommodate was unthinkable.

Basic training includes the clear message that there is no time for weakness or hesitation in doing what needs to be done. As the quotation that started this section describes, sharing or showing any vulnerability with your fellow soldiers—or with your family or friends back home—was not an option.

As veterans, many of us carry this mindset with us into civilian life, where we keep quiet about our struggles with physical, emotional, or social pain as a way to protect the people we care about. We don't want to be a burden to our family or other loved ones. We want to be strong for them, and we think we're putting their needs first by minimizing or denying our own.

Yet by concealing our pain, we may actually be inflicting pain on some of the important people in our lives. When we leave family members and friends out of this part of our life, they often feel misled or lied to. This can create misunderstandings, misinterpretations, misperceptions, and misconceptions about events and situations. It also creates confusion about how each person understands and values the relationship.

It's ironic, of course, that veterans are so often unwilling to allow others to help carry their burdens when they so selflessly do so for so many others. Can't this go both ways, where we give and take? As a group, veterans are defined by sacrificial service. We have repeatedly carried heavy loads for others. It's time to correct and change the mindset that keeps too many of us stuck and alone. It's time to let others help us.

We begin to do this when we share our experience and pain with our friends or loved ones. Letting others in might mean telling other veterans what we're going through. To get healthy and grow this skill, we may also benefit from the guidance of a counselor or therapist.

We also need to give our loved ones credit for their own strength. This includes our partners or spouses, our sisters and brothers, or sometimes our parents or nearest and dearest friends. In our work with veterans, we have found, with very few exceptions, that the people closest to them actually want to help. Veterans are most often met with reassurance that their sharing does not create a burden. Instead, opening up creates a deeper sense of closeness and trust in relationships.

Trusting a Significant Other

If you have a spouse or significant other person in your life, they can be a major support for dealing with pain—especially the social pains you experience. Having somebody this close to talk to, to trust, and to share with can reduce isolation and help you process feelings, experiences, and questions. Building a post-military life together can be a source of joy and shared purpose.

Opening up to receive these benefits from your partner can be difficult, of course. The last thing most of us want to do is place a burden on someone else—especially someone we love. The possibility of hurting your loved one by sharing your pain with them may feel like too big a risk. A big key to this problem is trust. In any relationship, trust is a quality that you build together. It takes time and practice.

As a veteran, you may have difficulty trusting yourself, other people, and the world in general. It can be hard to expect good things when you've experienced really hard ones, whether those hard times happened before, during, or after your time in the military. These difficulties with trust may be affecting your ability and willingness to share your feelings, stories, or the full extent of your pain with others, especially with your significant other.

Trusting that your spouse or significant other can handle the weight of the physical, emotional, and social pains you endure while still loving and caring for you may seem difficult to imagine. The fact is your spouse or significant other might not respond in the way you fear. It's more likely they've been waiting for you to share, and they're ready to help or support you.

So how do you accept this idea and develop trust? As usual, the first step is the scariest. You must take the risk of opening up. Think about how you decided that your brother or sister in your unit had your back. You got into a shitty situation, and they demonstrated to you that they were trustworthy—that they could handle whatever was going on. You could trust their strength and competence. You could trust that they cared about you.

The same thing applies to your loved one. They won't know what you don't tell them. It can feel counterintuitive, but letting your partner in on your pain helps heal—both you and them.

We cannot assume that our loved one understands us just because they are nearby or we live under the same roof. Trust and communication are the core elements of connection and understanding, and these are what make our primary relationships work best and grow stronger. A loved one can empathize in a way that is supportive and nonjudgmental, but this can't happen unless you let them.

CHECKPOINT:

- Choose three words that might describe a close relationship in which you felt comfortable enough to ask for support. Which of your current relationships are like this?

- What has made trusting others difficult for you in the past? How did you overcome that difficulty?
- How do you try and show others that you are worthy of their trust?

Our Military Family
—

Humans are born with the instinct to connect with other people. In the military, this urge attaches itself to the people you depend on for support and mutual care: your battle buddies. These connections were probably even stronger if you deployed or served in a hardship tour that allowed you little or no access to your family or friends at home. For some veterans, their fellow soldiers provided the only social connection during the entire length of service in the armed forces. This deep intimacy builds unit cohesion in the field, but it can also create a unique problem when soldiers go home.

What happens when you no longer have immediate access to the people who know you so well? What happens when you can't walk down the hall and talk with your closest friends about something that is bothering you?

You might say, "I would call them" or, "I would go visit them," but do you do this? Most veterans report that they don't. Many veterans have difficulty reaching out to anyone when they need help, whether it be to their closest battle buddies, other veterans, non-veteran friends, family members, or health care providers.

Given how close many veterans were to the people they served with, how come we struggle to connect with our close military friends and other battle buddies now that we're home? For some of us, the simple answer is distance. Veterans come from all walks of life and each corner of the country. Over the course of time, we lose track of where people are and the distances involved cause us to lose contact.

Wasn't that a nice bullshit answer? Here's the truth.

Veterans often entered the military at a young age. Many had not even started pursuing life's great accomplishments such as getting a good-paying job, getting married, having children, buying a boat (perhaps this is just a Minnesota thing), starting a small business, or pursuing some other dream.

When asked why and how they lost touch with their former friends and comrades, most veterans simply say, "Life happened." Following the life chapter that included their military service, and through no fault of their own, the basic business of making a living and working toward their goals meant they lost touch and grew apart. This is common and normal.

There is something to the answer about distance, of course. We most easily connect with those who are physically closest to us. Relationships that involve proximity take precedence. It's normal to come home and try to re-establish a support system with the people who are physically nearby—usually family and close friends. But this doesn't mean you no longer care for your battle buddies or that they don't care for you. We've observed that some veterans continue to have deep connection with their veteran friends whenever they are able to catch up—almost like time stood still. We seem to start again right where we left off.

Let's also acknowledge the common and powerful dynamic that affects our willingness and ability to reach out to veteran friends. This may be hard for you to hear or admit. Many veterans lose touch with their veteran counterparts because of fear. We're afraid of being the one whose life isn't going well. We don't want to be the one struggling and in need of help. We fear not being able to connect anymore, scared that we have nothing in common. We're afraid of not being as important to our friends as we once were. These thoughts are valid, yet they're also likely preventing you from reaching out and getting the connection and support you desperately need and want.

How come we let fear control us? We depended on our veteran family for years. We depended on our family before the military for years prior to that. Yet, many veterans feel disconnected from both groups after returning home. Did we change? Did they change? Is it pride? Is it ego?

Every veteran who reads this likely has a different answer or combination of answers to these questions, and that's okay. But what if the tables were flipped, and your battle buddy was the one experiencing the pain of disconnection from their family, friends, coworkers, or fellow veterans? We can almost guarantee you would say, "Reach out!"

How come the rules are different for them? Is it okay for them to reach out, but not acceptable for you to do the same? Come on! Nobody can know what's going on for you unless you tell them. This includes our military family as well as the family, friends, and significant others we came home to.

It's okay to depend on others, and it is courageous to let someone know about the challenges you're experiencing and how they're affecting you. If you're not okay, tell someone. If you're doing well, share that too. You were able to ask for help and depend on others in the military, and you provided support to your buddies at the same time. You have those muscles. You can find ways to let these strengths continue to work in your life as a veteran.

Tangible Next Steps
—

Let Go of Comparisons
Take a second to ask yourself to whom or to what you tend to compare yourself. Are you trying to keep up with the younger person you once were? Are you measuring yourself against memories or ideas of people you once admired or looked up to? Are these comparisons fair? What feels important or helpful about looking

at yourself in this way? Are you mad or sad that you can't accomplish something you want or need? You might choose to reflect on these questions in your journal or go over them with a trusted friend or therapist, or revisit them at a later time.

Letting go of comparisons often starts with understanding how this way of thinking serves you. Finding out the "why" you behave or think in certain ways can help you better determine "how to" move on from the past and focus on the here and now. Grounding yourself in the present reality might mean writing a list of all the things in your current life that you're grateful for. It might include telling someone a story about a time in your life when you learned something new, started an important relationship, or changed for the better. Accept that life experiences are going to impact you. You're a different person than you were, and you will be a different person as you grow and change.

"Right-Size" Your Expectations

When our expectations for others, for situations, or for ourselves aren't met, many of us become disappointed or even embittered. This can have both a direct and an indirect impact on our willingness to trust or our ability to hope. For example, if you had expectations to receive ongoing support and care after you left the military and those expectations have not been met, you may feel abandoned or let down by the government (directly). Or maybe you feel abandoned by certain family members or friends who have not been there for you in ways that you had expected.

Reflecting on your expectations of what the military and other people and institutions owe you may be important for you. Ask yourself how reasonable your expectations are. If after careful review, you determine that your expectations might be too high or too low, adjust them to a size that feels more appropriate or realistic. Whenever we take this kind of personal inventory, we're better prepared to understand the ways our expectations affect our sense of belonging and connection.

Make a List of People You Can Count On

Throughout this book you've heard us say "Reach out," "Talk," or "Connect." Maybe this idea still feels abstract or uncertain for you. Let's get concrete. Take the time right now to list five people you believe are willing and able to support you. This can include close friends and family members, members of your military family, or people like pastors or rabbis or other religious leaders—even former coaches or teachers. If you're working with a therapist or have a Twelve Step sponsor, that person could be on your list as well.

Write down their names or the way you think of them (e.g., "My sister," "James," "battle buddy"). Then write down the means by which you can contact them. Are they accessible to you via phone, email, or social media?

Next, reach out to these individuals to simply let them know they're on your list. This will give them a chance to confirm that they're willing and able to offer you this kind of support. Explain exactly when or how you will contact them. Will you regularly call on a certain day of the week or time of day? Will it be whenever you're feeling a certain way, such as when you're happy, mad, sad, anxious, or celebrating a big accomplishment? You may choose to write down this plan for reaching out in your journal or the notes section on your phone. This can also just be a mental note for yourself.

Once you've built your list and developed your plan, use it.

Stop Taking Things Personally

For many veterans, this tangible next step involves an internal dialogue. Begin by imagining that a civilian asks you a question or makes a comment and you find yourself getting offended or simply pissed off. Can you picture it? Before you imagine the response you'd give, stop. In this moment try asking yourself, *How come I feel offended?* Then ask yourself, *Could this person's comment or question be a way in which they're trying to connect with me or better understand me or my experiences?*

We get to choose how we respond to everyone and everything. This includes moments when we feel offended. Instead of feeling personally attacked by the person's words and then responding in an angry manner, or perhaps not responding at all (we're pretty good at giving the cold shoulder), try answering a question with a question. Say, for example, "What makes you ask that?" or "How come you ask that question?" Getting curious about what may be behind certain statements or questions can help you not take someone else's comments personally.

Most people aren't assholes (you may have to trust us on this); they just want to better understand or to connect. Exploring the reasons someone may be asking a question or making a comment will help you learn more about the person and their intentions. You'll also learn more about yourself, including how or in what ways some questions or comments irritate you.

Conserve Your Energy

If you find yourself in survival mode (i.e., the "fight, flight, or freeze" crisis response), try and ask yourself if this feeling is appropriate for the situation you're facing. Do you find yourself responding to a situation in a manner that is the same size as the problem at hand? Survival mode responses are often overreactions.

Here are a few examples:

- Lee gets into a blow-out fight with her spouse about the lights being left on in the house.
- After an argument with a friend, Jayson leaves the house right at his kids' bedtime to go for a long drive by himself.

- Riley freezes up after a tough incident with his kids and won't share his feelings with his spouse.

When you recognize such extreme reactions in yourself, try taking a breath and telling yourself you can respond differently. This will conserve your energy.

There are some situations that warrant higher energy responses, but most don't. If you have trouble determining this, try listing a few of the problems you may be experiencing in your life right now. You can do this in a journal or somewhere else. Separate your list into "big problems" and "small problems." Then look at the lists. Items on the "big problems" list may warrant a survival mode response, but often many of the big problems still don't warrant this large of a reaction. Ask yourself, *Are there any items that actually deserve a survival mode response? How come?*

When you do notice yourself putting enormous energy into everyday interactions that may not require so much energy, try and step it down or redirect. Try to do this by catching yourself and rethinking your behavior. You may decide to pause a conversation or decide to try something else to help you relax.

The only time you need to respond in a survival mode manner is when crisis-level problems appear. Otherwise, you can conserve your energy. Learning how to identify and let go of smaller problems will bring more mental space and time into your life and allow you to feel more relaxed.

Check In with Your Primary Relationships

As you begin to practice sharing and feel more comfortable doing so (and we hope this book helps you), check in with your spouse or significant other. Ask them about their feelings related to your time in the military and their experience with your communication about this part of your life. These relationships are places where closeness, openness, trust, and communication are deeply important—but those things don't happen automatically.

You may find that opening this door offers you a chance to reminisce about your shared experience. Your questions may also reveal how your significant other felt or is feeling after learning more about your experience. Talk about these feelings together and about how they affect your relationship.

After this conversation, spend some time reflecting on what you heard. What have you learned about closeness or trust or communication? You might process this internally by writing or just thinking about it or externally by discussing the experience with your spouse or significant other. If you're not used to talking about your military experience with your loved one, that's okay. This may be something that you need to work up to. Initiate these conversations at your own pace when you feel ready.

Don't Make an Ass out of You (or Me)

As we discussed in this chapter, assumptions are dangerous! They can cause social pain on their own or turn simple awkwardness into something even more uncomfortable. We don't like when others make judgments about us as veterans, so we shouldn't make judgments about those who don't share our experience. Remember, too, that assumptions and first impressions are often incorrect. Nothing can replace the experience of actually getting to know someone. Of course, this can be difficult—especially when it comes to disclosure—but it's something you can do at your own pace. Meeting others as real people with complex experiences (just like ours) can help us avoid jumping to conclusions or making assumptions.

The more people we find whom we can connect with, the less isolated we will feel. Allowing others into our lives and our stories can help ease the social pain we may be experiencing as veterans.

CHAPTER SIX

—

Pain and Addiction

> *The military has a culture that is steeped in alcohol. Work hard, play hard. We can't drink while we are underway, so when we pulled into port, most of us (myself included) got very drunk. This helped us with the loneliness of being away from our families, helped us blow off some steam.*
>
> **—EMILY, US COAST GUARD**

IN THE SUMMER OF 1945, people celebrated the end of World War II in all kinds of ways. There are many well-known pictures of this moment in history. One example is of a sailor and woman kissing. Others include gigantic crowds celebrating in the streets of London and Paris, and in New York City's Times Square. What these photos do not depict is the vast amount of alcohol that was consumed during this time as people all across the globe celebrated the end of the deadliest conflict in human history.

Within both military and veteran communities, the use and abuse of alcohol is widespread. In addition to celebration, alcohol gets used to calm down or lower anxiety, to cope with physical pain, to numb feelings of emotional pain such as grief, and to pass the time with friends and family. Alcohol is often part of social gatherings where veterans and service members remember fallen friends and reminisce about their experiences.

And we don't just drink. Research and clinical data have found veterans use marijuana, cocaine and other stimulants (including Adderall and Ritalin), nicotine, and opioids (including heroin), as well as alcohol.[1] Veterans also use substances like methamphetamine, hashish, LSD and other hallucinogens, and various prescription medications. A recent study found that 11 percent of veterans seeking help at the VA for the first time likely met criteria for substance use disorder.[2] If you don't currently have a problem with substances, it's likely that you know a veteran who does. You're probably also aware of how addiction can end careers, ruin lives, and destroy families.

Using alcohol or other drugs isn't the only coping strategy with an addictive component that veterans use to suppress or escape physical, emotional, and social pain. Addictive behaviors including gambling and compulsive sexual behavior as well as disordered eating are unfortunately part of many veterans' toolkits for dealing with pain of all sorts.

Addictive substances and behaviors have become pain management gear for a staggering number of veterans. This chapter will describe and explore some of these unhealthy coping tools and explain how they can become go-to strategies, both by themselves and in combination. We'll also briefly outline how addiction works, describe how some of us are more susceptible to it than others, and discuss connections between addiction and mental health. Finally, we'll discuss what you can do if you're worried about your own relationship with addictive substances or behaviors. Along the way and at the end of the chapter, we'll offer suggestions for what you can do if you're concerned about your own use of substances when it comes to dealing (or not dealing) with your pain.

Substances and the Military

In the military community, soldiers have had a long-standing tradition of using substances to relax, celebrate, or simply combat boredom. Substances were actually issued as gear for decades. During World War II, soldiers' rations included cartons of cigarettes, which were either smoked or traded and bartered among soldiers and the civilians they were stationed nearby. It was not until 1975 that the military stopped including cigarettes in rations for soldiers.

It is likely that you or a buddy may have smoked cigarettes or used chewing tobacco while in the military, whether you were on breaks, waiting for formation to start, immediately following a mission or activity, or even while driving on a mission. You may have even lit up a cigarette right after a 10K run. Woof!

There is a similar relationship between alcohol and the military. Alcohol is widely available on bases, most of which also feature clubs or bars to drink in. During the most recent military conflicts, alcohol was shipped in on pallets for soldiers catching some R&R or a break from the front lines. Throughout history, alcohol has been widely used to celebrate military victories and to "heal" wounds of loss and sorrow.

In his book *The Things They Carried,* Tim O'Brien paints a picture of his time in the Vietnam War.[3] He uses the metaphor of a soldier's possessions to examine the "things" they carried with them during the war and ultimately into their lives beyond their experience in Vietnam. O'Brien describes physical things such as lighters, weapons, and socks his buddies carried but also memories and mental and psychological experiences that stayed with them, such as guilt, shame, worry, and fear. Some of the soldiers described in the book kept and used cigarettes, tranquilizers, and marijuana. These substances were often used to ease physical pain and lighten the emotional loads they carried. For many soldiers, substances became a normal part of their gear or pack.

A common experience for soldiers is the fear that you are missing something before you head out on a mission or exercise. This includes equipment, of course—nobody wants to be in the field needing something they forgot to pack. It also often includes a substance of some kind.

When a soldier discovers that a substance takes away pain, subdues fear, numbs feeling, or even improves functioning, it cements its place on the preparation list for the next mission. For many veterans, the fear of not having a shot of vodka, not taking a quick puff of marijuana, or not smoking their lucky cigarette before a major event is stress inducing. Humans enjoy consistency. Military people *love* consistency.

While in the military, many of you likely found substances or other addictive habits or processes to be an essential part of the gear you felt you needed to survive. It may have become second nature for you to simply pat your pants or jacket pocket to make sure your substance was there, ready to go, whenever it was needed. For some veterans, the feeling of not having the right gear, the right coping skill, or the right support is a life-or-death-type feeling.

Some of us would rather have the wrong gear, such as alcohol, drugs, or sex, than no gear at all. Most gear initially fits (that is, it works) but even when it stops being as effective as it once was, we hold on to it. For too many of us, alcohol and drug use is a piece of gear that became difficult to turn in when the mission of military service ended.

CHECKPOINT:
- When it comes to the "gear" of alcohol, tobacco, or other drugs, what gear did you take with you from your time in the military?
- When was the first time, if any, that you used substances to not feel a feeling or emotion? Did it work? For how long?
- What would you like to change about your substance use?

The Gear You Brought with You

—

> *I used drugs as a sort of rebellious escape before joining the Army, and in my first few years in the Army, I would use alcohol to sort of fit in. It wasn't until I started deploying and experiencing combat that I started abusing alcohol as a way to escape and cope with my feelings.*
>
> —**JIM, US ARMY**

Our relationship with substance use prior to the military often set the stage for how and why we drank or used drugs while we served. These patterns can also continue into our lives as veterans.

If you grew up in a family where one or more members had an addiction to alcohol or other drugs, you're more likely to also have trouble managing or controlling your use of substances. This is not automatic, of course. Some people who grow up with multiple risk factors for addiction don't have any issues with substance use throughout their adult lives. That's because addiction results from a combination of factors. These include our genes, where and how we were raised, and our own behavior around substances—such as whether we use alcohol or other drugs as gear to fit in or cope with stress and pain.

One way that drinking, using drugs, or misusing prescription medication may have appeared to help us before the military was in managing our mental health. Using substances to subdue, numb, or ignore intense emotions or negative feelings like anxiety or fear is usually something learned by watching or listening to others. Some veterans describe having a parent who wouldn't talk about their feelings, for example, but would drink or use in front of them while trying to manage a difficult life situation or manage these feelings. These examples of how to manage life stressors may come from other family members and friends as well.

Here's a common story that illustrates how many of us developed our early relationships with substances.

Imagine you are a sixteen-year-old high school student. You have started to dabble in using alcohol and cannabis or pills. Mostly it's limited to weekends, when you party with your friends and other kids—sometimes competing to see how much you can consume before throwing up or passing out. Sometimes you drink until you black out. Luckily, your hangovers aren't that bad. Occasionally you drink when you're all by yourself and you find that having a few beers or smoking a bowl makes you feel less anxious.

Most of us can relate to stories like this. The teenager's use might seem rather harmless; the negative effects appear minimal. Getting drunk or high as a teenager almost feels like a rite of passage.

But what are the underlying unhealthy assumptions that a young person may take away from these experiences?

Kids in these circumstances might come to believe the following:

- Using substances is a normal way to connect with others.
- Substance use is a fun game that can involve competition.
- Using substances can help you feel better when you're bored, sad or depressed, lonely, anxious, or frustrated.

Let's note right away that we do not endorse these takeaways! These and similar beliefs have been and continue to provide a basis for all kinds of unhealthy and damaging behaviors that destroy lives, ruin relationships, and end careers. That being said, it's not hard to see how these beliefs form and how they can stick with us into adulthood.

Chances are you acquired some substance-related gear like this before you entered the military. The ideas, beliefs, and rules about when and how to use alcohol and drugs we picked up and used as young people may have followed us into the service. For many, the culture you experienced in the military either reinforced these rules or expected you to adopt different ones.

CHECKPOINT:

- What lessons were part of your early substance use "education" as a teenager or young adult?
- Which of these messages were part of the military culture you experienced?
- How did your military service change the way you used substances? How did your use become gear that differs from what you came in with?
- Which pieces of your substance use gear are you still trying to use in your pain-relief mission as a veteran?

Addiction—How Optional Gear Becomes Essential

———

Coming from a very high tempo, operating in the yellow as the Navy would put it, I didn't have the ability to cope with fifteen months of mental strain. What I used to cope was drinking copious amounts of alcohol. We would wake up in the morning and go to first formation. After, we would all go directly to the barracks and drink. This continued on for years as my coping mechanism. As my main coping mechanism, I would drink a ton during any stressful event.

—RUSSELL, US NAVY

The fields of medicine, addiction, and addiction recovery have come a long way in the last one hundred years. Alcoholics Anonymous was founded in 1935; Narcotics Anonymous in 1953. Over the course of human history, medical science has developed thousands of theories about what addiction is and what contributes to its development. Some believed it was a purely psychological thing. Others believed it was physical. Still others argued it was cultural or an issue for a certain type of person.

Today, addiction is understood and treated as a disease that includes and affects both the mind and body. It's described as a dysfunction of certain parts of the brain, like the reward system. We can be genetically predisposed to addiction. Like many other diseases, it can be chronic, which means it persists throughout a person's life. Most addiction experts also believe that the disease is progressive—that it will continue to worsen until we get help. Addiction can be treated, but so far there's no cure.

Genetic predisposition means that some of us are more likely to become addicted because of factors we inherited from our ancestors, along with other characteristics, like the color of our eyes or the shape of our hands or how tall we are. A metaphor may help. Imagine there are one million light switches inside your body. These switches control your susceptibility to addiction. Some of these light switches are already turned on when you are born due to genetics—they're more hardwired—while others get flipped on when you experience a certain kind of event, such as childhood trauma or chronic physical pain. Some of these switches get activated by using substances early in life. If you drank heavily in high school or misused Adderall to cram for tests, you are more likely to become addicted to substances in later life.

In addition to these risk factors, addiction involves a psychological process of reinforcement. Human beings learn by doing. If we try a certain behavior (such as drinking alcohol) and get a positive or enjoyable outcome (our physical, emotional, or social pain is reduced or goes away), we're more likely to repeat the behavior. Reinforcement also works the other way. When we do something that immediately (and repeatedly) produces a negative or unlikable outcome, we're more likely to avoid doing that thing.

You may be wondering, *Well, what happens when I realize that what I thought was helping me is actually bad for me?* This is the paradoxical problem at the core of addiction. People who have an addiction to a substance often know that their drinking or using is creating negative outcomes in their life but they feel unable to stop. This inability to change behavior is caused by a change that's happened in our brains from repeated substance use. Addiction hijacks our ability to stop drinking or using—even when we know the substances that once seemed to help us are now harming us.

Reinforcement can also make stopping feel impossible. If someone is using alcohol daily, for example, and abruptly stops, they will enter serious withdrawal. A few common symptoms of alcohol withdrawal include shaking, sweating, increased heart rate, unbearable anxiety, and tremors. Naturally, we do not want to feel like this. One quick way to stop these symptoms is to drink again. This creates a reinforcement loop that our brains learn. Now the brain and body send the message that if we stop using, we'll suffer and the only way to keep these negative symptoms at bay is to keep using.

At this point, addiction has taken hold. We're no longer able to control our choice to use. Instead, we're in a vicious cycle of maintaining or self-medicating with a substance to survive. The "optional gear" once used to celebrate with friends or as a remedy for grief becomes an essential part of getting through every day.

Veterans and Substance Use

Picture yourself at a military ball. You're dressed in your Class A uniform and sitting beside your buddies. You're reminiscing about good times, drinks in hand, and mentally preparing yourself to stand up and get your glass filled from the grog (for those who have not had the pleasure—or displeasure—of drinking from a grog, imagine a combination of alcoholic spirits, including but not limited to vodka, bourbon, tequila, and/or gin, which ends up tasting like straight diesel fuel). As you walk outside, you see a vast number of soldiers of all ranks smoking cigarettes. It almost looks like a factory just produced its next item and the furnace turned on.

There are two takeaways from this mental picture: One, grogs are gross, and they're an unfortunate tradition within military settings. Two, it's quite common for veterans to become addicted to more than one substance, such as alcohol and nicotine. This creates two sets of cravings, two sets of reinforcement behaviors, two sets of withdrawals, and one gigantic problem that is not easy to shake without help.

Some of us entered the military already struggling with substance use issues; others started misusing substances while in the military. Some veterans did not touch alcohol or drugs until long after leaving the military but have since developed a full-fledged substance use disorder. There are also large numbers of veterans who do not struggle with substances. This section is for the many of you who do.

What Veterans Use

As explored earlier in the chapter, the most common addictive substance used by members of the military and veterans is alcohol. Tobacco is another leading candidate; many veterans started smoking or dipping while in the military. It is not uncommon to see both addictions together.

Though not endorsed or tolerated for recreational use, the military has prescribed or supplied other addictive substances to its members to address medical and mental health issues. When used as intended, these substances and medications can be remarkably helpful. Widespread and prolonged reliance on these drugs, however, has led many to develop ongoing problems with addiction. The most common of these substances are opioid medications and benzodiazepines. The combination of the two can also be very dangerous.

Opioids for Physical Pain

As we noted in chapter 3, addiction to opioids has become a big problem in the United States, both inside and outside the military. Opioids include fentanyl, heroin, hydrocodone, codeine, oxycodone, and morphine. Some opioids are prescribed; others are illegal.

Using strong medications to combat acute pain has a long military tradition. In World War II, soldiers were rationed a morphine pack that was to be used to relieve pain if they were injured. Medics would mark wounded soldiers with an "M" on their forehead to ensure the next medical professional knew they had received a shot of morphine.

We have a human instinct to help or relieve someone who is in pain, and opioid medications can be remarkable tools for doing that. These drugs continue to have a medical use within the military.

However, the easy availability of opioid pain medication has led to widespread use and misuse both inside and outside the military. Individuals who become addicted to opioids often have some common stories. For example, some veterans develop an addiction while taking opioid prescription medications for past and/or current chronic physical pain. Other veterans may begin using opioids because they enjoy the feeling of numbness they produce, or they may simply be experimenting with drugs.

The use of opioids is also attractive to veterans for a deeper reason. We were taught to always be "mission ready." This imperative created and reinforced a value system that required us to be strong, be available at a moment's notice, and show no pain. Opioids can produce those effects. If you have a sore back, an opioid may relieve it quickly, if temporarily, allowing you to accomplish your mission.

Unfortunately, because these powerful drugs mimic the naturally occurring pain blockers in our bodies, we can easily get used to these effects and begin to rely on opioids. Over time and with repeated use, we can develop an addiction that is difficult, but not impossible, to combat.

We also recognize that not all individuals who have taken opioids for an extended period of time intended to do so and not all fit into the "addiction" category. In fact, oftentimes, individuals have developed something different than an addiction to their medication called "dependence." Dependence is when the body is relying on a substance to produce a certain effect. Being dependent on medications to help with ongoing pain is a slippery slope due to tolerance issues and addiction issues. Tolerance is when someone receives a reduced level of relief from a usual dose of a substance.

Stopping opioid use needs to involve your doctor's help. Together you can develop a medication taper plan. This will include a scheduled reduction of medications that incrementally and gradually occurs over time in a safe manner. Opioid withdrawal can be dangerous, with seriously uncomfortable symptoms. Depending on how long you've been taking the drug and how high your usual dose has been, it can take months to safely lower your dose.

Reducing your reliance on opioids is a challenge, but you can rise to it. Success will require you to enlist the support of your prescribing doctor, your health care team, and the people you care about. Together, you can devise a plan, manage your symptoms, and develop alternative ways to cope with pain.

HELP FOR OPIOID ADDICTION

If you need immediate help for an opioid addiction or are ready to stop relying on these medications to manage your pain, contact your health care professional. The VA also has a crisis line.

Call 988 or 1-800-273-TALK (8255) and choose option 1, or text 838255. Also visit www.va.gov for further resources.

Benzodiazepines for Anxiety and Pain

One of the most common mental health diagnoses for veterans and service members is anxiety disorders. Anxiety might feel like worrying excessively and sometimes for no reason, feeling on edge, having a hard time concentrating on things or tasks, difficulty sleeping (either falling or staying asleep), irritability (including outbursts of anger), and tension in your muscles. If you experience some of these symptoms and they get in your way of doing what you want to do, you might have some anxiety.

Anxiety among veterans has some distinct characteristics. In our experience, veterans with anxiety often feel an added sense of hypervigilance or uneasiness along with the more common symptoms described above. It can feel like an energy that's hard to escape or get rid of. This restless energy could be connected to the military culture of *go-go-go*. It can also reflect a deep-seated need to assert control over your environment in order to feel safe. Veteran-related anxiety is real and can be powerfully debilitating. A common anti-anxiety tool used in health care settings is psychotropic medication.

Enter benzodiazepines.

Like opioids, benzodiazepine medications can be appropriate to use in certain situations and times for some veterans. Also known as "benzos," these drugs are a type of sedative often prescribed to treat severe anxiety. They may also be used as a triage medication for panic attacks. Common benzos include Xanax, Valium, Ativan, and Klonopin. These medications offer what's called an "all-system effect." They offer an immediate, whole-body, sedative, or even tranquilizing relief.

Great! Good-bye panic attack!

Or is it that great?

Because they work so well, it can be really easy to rely on these medications to feel calm, "normal," at ease, or content without trying alternative, healthy, more sustainable options. Having a medication do the work appears to decrease or even eliminate the need for the veteran to use other coping skills to manage anxiety symptoms. But what happens when we are 100 percent reliant on this medication to manage everyday challenges? What happens when we begin to rely on it to simply function? Veterans can find themselves in a horrible situation when their prescriber realizes they've become dependent or addicted and the provider decides to stop prescribing the medication. Benzodiazepine withdrawal is no joke—it can even be lethal if not done correctly.

In addition to the problems that come with reliance on medications, benzodiazepines can make it difficult for individuals to learn new tasks or take on new information. Here is an example of what this might look like. Let's picture Susan. Susan is afraid of flying on an airplane due to her experiences in the military, so she asks her provider for Xanax to help with her next trip. She takes the Xanax and all goes as planned; Susan gets through her anxiety-provoking flight experience. However, Susan now assumes she has to take this medication every time she flies. You can see how this practice can quickly develop into a reliance on the medication. The benzodiazepine offers Susan a quick fix. It helps "take away" her anxiety in the situation and allows her to make it through the flight, but it also blocks her ability to learn that she can get through the stressful experience with her own coping.

If Susan were to pair her medication with other tools such as listening to music, distracting herself with an adult coloring book, and deep breathing/sensory strategies, she may be able to reduce or completely stop her benzodiazepine use.

Individuals with chronic pain may also use the all-system effects of benzodiazepines to help relieve their physical pain. Though they may provide some relief from pain, this is not what these medications are intended for.

When individuals are using a benzodiazepine to address their physical pain, they may also have an opioid on board. This is when we get into especially dangerous waters. Opioids and benzodi-azepines together can have a major impact on your respiratory system, slowing things down significantly. This is something many individuals may feel "they have experience with" and "know their bodies," but the fact is that no one can predict how this combina-tion can impact you each time, and there are many outside factors (your environment, stress, sleep, hydration, etc.) that can make this combination extremely dangerous and potentially lethal. Overall, benzodiazepines may have a role to play in helping vet-erans manage crises or anxiety-provoking situations, but over time and with consistent use, these medications may be more harmful than helpful.

If you're currently regularly using benzodiazepines to manage anxiety, talk to your prescriber about a plan to possibly reduce your use of this medication. Your plan may include looking into non-benzodiazepine options for anxiety. Consider adding some of the relaxation strategies we offer in this book, especially the breath-ing and sensory techniques that were included in chapter 3. Don't stop taking your medication on your own, however. Like stopping opioids, getting off benzos can trigger severe withdrawal symp-toms. Doing this safely requires coordination with your health care provider. Remember, though, that as tough as it may seem, it is possible to get off benzos. With help, you can break free from the hold substances have on your life.

Mental Health and Addiction

Many people who have a substance use disorder or other addiction also struggle with mental health concerns. When these issues show up together and the person is diagnosed with both a substance use disorder and a mental health disorder, they are said to have "co-occurring disorders."

Common mental health concerns many veterans face while also dealing with addiction include anxiety, panic attacks, mood-related disorders including depression and bipolar disorder, trauma-related disorders such as PTSD, disordered eating, self-harm and suicidality, and obsessive-compulsive disorder. For some, mental health symptoms are only present when using substances like alcohol. Perhaps you only get sad or reminisce about painful memories when drinking heavily, for example. Or maybe you get anxious when you are around a lot of other people while sober, so you drink to feel better. Maybe your anxiety goes down. This is an example of how your addiction is talking to your mental health and vice versa.

Because of their cultural values, defense mechanisms, and life experiences, veterans often deal with unique forms of loss, grief, trauma, anxiety, and depression. Moreover, veterans learn to use substances such as alcohol as ways to cope, push down, and "heal" wounds. This is often reinforced by cultural expectations, which can create a unique storm for both addiction and mental health as co-occurring concerns.

Co-occurring disorders often have a direct influence on one another. If one is being managed effectively, the other may be better regulated as well. For example, if a veteran struggles with anxiety and knows that their anxiety is a trigger to drink alcohol, efforts to manage their anxiety might reduce the risk of alcohol use.

Another unique mental health situation many veterans face involves the emotional effects of addiction to pain medication because of a long-fought battle with chronic physical pain. Many veterans entered the military at a young age, perhaps eighteen years old, but when they left the military, they felt like they—or at least their knees and back—were already forty. Now those veterans require a pill to simply survive the day and move from point A to point B. When a person feels dependent on something such as a pill, it can create feelings of shame, guilt, or sadness. Enter depression. Suddenly, we have addiction, chronic pain, and mental health talking to one another. Veterans deal with co-occurring disorders throughout much of their lives, and it is important to understand how each issue interacts with and influences the other. The more awareness you have about the co-occurring issues you may be experiencing, the more likely you are to find a way to better manage them.

Do You Have a Problem?

It's very common to use alcohol and drugs to alleviate minor pain, to relieve boredom, or to feel excited or confident in social settings. These substances are a kind of coping tool. Because they tend to mask problems and reduce symptoms of pain and discomfort rather than address and resolve the causes of physical, emotional, or social pain, they often function as defense mechanisms. In addition to allowing you to avoid learning and using more healthy coping strategies, drugs and alcohol are addictive. This makes them dangerous. If you ask a friend who identifies as an alcoholic or drug addict, they will likely tell you that the progression from substance use to substance misuse to addiction can happen quickly and seem invisible.

As noted earlier, addiction (substance use disorder) is a disease, not a choice. The disease causes people to have difficulty controlling their use of substances. If you use alcohol or drugs to feel good, especially when you are feeling bad or down and want to feel better, you may have a problem on your hands. If you use alcohol or drugs to numb, ignore or forget, avoid or stuff, release, or displace your pain, you may have a problem on your hands. If you use alcohol or drugs to lower the severity of mental health symptoms, such as anxiety or depression, you may have a problem on your hands.

COMMON SYMPTOMS OF SUBSTANCE USE DISORDER

- You experience an increasing urge to use drugs or drink alcohol.
- You are unable to stop drinking or using drugs, even when it leads to unwelcome outcomes.
- Your drinking or drug use causes changes to your primary relationships.
- You feel sad, regretful, depressed, or anxious about your level of drinking or drug use.
- You get sick or experience symptoms of withdrawal whenever you try to stop drinking or using.
- It takes more and more alcohol or stronger doses of the drug to get you drunk or high.[4]

If you have told yourself that your use of substances or your reliance on compulsive behaviors like sex or exercise or gambling is "not that bad," even while worrying that it might be, you're likely aware of two things. One, you know that these things can lead to further pain and complications. Two, you're open to exploring whether your use or behavior is causing problems in your life. This is a good thing! Getting a substance use assessment will help you evaluate your current level of use and your risk for addiction. This will give you more information about your options for dealing with it. Treating addiction can include inpatient or outpatient treatment programs, peer support groups like AA or NA, and individual counseling.

One of the foundational steps in many substance treatment programs is recognizing that there is a problem. Whether we're talking about the reality of our pain or the facts about our substance use, if we don't name or acknowledge the truth of what we're facing and how it's affecting us, we run the risk of continuing to go on like nothing's wrong. But all the while we're suffering—and slowly watching ourselves fail to live our lives the way we want to. Hiding problems with substance use brings its own kind of pain—often experienced as an unbearable blend of physical discomfort, emotional agony, and social isolation.

If your substance use is adding to your pain, if you are experiencing any of the symptoms of substance use disorder, or if you suspect you might be an addict or alcoholic, please know you are not alone.

If your eyes got laser focused by that last sentence, this paragraph is speaking directly to you. Give an AA or NA meeting a try; in many areas, you can even find a veteran-specific AA or NA meeting. In Twelve Step programs, the only requirement to attend a meeting is having a desire to stop drinking or using. These groups are completely anonymous. There's no registration process, no fee, no appointment to make, and no pressure to conform to any particular belief.

You can also find help by talking with your primary care doctor or a therapist who has expertise in veterans' issues. Or you can go directly to an addiction treatment center or even a hospital. And you can always call a buddy or tell a member of your family what you are dealing with. Talk. Talk. Talk. Many veterans are shocked when they discover how many other veterans struggle with addiction. The only way to find support is to let somebody in.

Let's close by giving you massive credit for what you likely have already done or tried to do to find relief from your pain. We are dead serious here. Veterans are some of the most creative, strong, compassionate, badass, and caring people in the world. We will do anything for others. We will protect others. However, we do not always do as well when it comes to caring for, helping, and protecting ourselves, but we have to! If your use of substances as coping tools has begun to threaten your health, safety, and happiness, it's time to get help.

Tangible Next Steps

———

Change Your Gear

Consider whether you have been using substances such as drugs and alcohol to deal with your pain. Maybe these have been part of your go-to gear for a while. That makes sense! It really does. We bet it was probably very effective for a while—that using a substance did help you feel better about something happening in your life or that it helped you avoid feeling anything at all. But is it still as effective? Are you using substances to subdue or numb painful feelings, thoughts, or memories? Let's be real, did those problems or feelings go away after using? Or are you using substances now because you can't stop and now you have a whole new problem?

Whatever your answer is, know that substances are bad, dysfunctional, recall-worthy, maladaptive, tainted, shit pieces of gear. It's time to retire this tool and find other and better ways to cope with your pain. Addiction to drugs and alcohol is a disease. We acknowledge that suggesting you change out your gear is a big ask. However, knowing when our gear is faulty and becoming willing to adopt more effective gear or tools is how we can achieve the changes we want for our future.

Expand Your Packing List

If you use substances to subdue pain, you probably picked up this gear before, during, or shortly after your time in the military. Think of this as part of the gear you were rationed or assigned. Excessive drinking is part of military culture. It may have helped you celebrate, fit in, find friends, or express emotion. It may have helped you endure unimaginable pain, suffering, and loss. But at some point, it's going to start hurting more than it helps. Maybe that's already the case for you.

So try something else. When we have one coping tool that worked or works, such as relying on substances, we hold back from using others. Most of us take the path of least resistance and ignore alternative or complementary options. Here is our challenge to you. Start a running list of other, healthier ways you could cope with your pain instead of using drugs or alcohol, or misusing prescribed medication. Shoot for a list of 100! Maybe start with the Tangible Next Steps in this book to help come up with your own personalized gear that you think will work for you.

Develop a New Type of Tolerance

Just like Susan in the example about her fear of flying, we generally don't like dealing with discomfort. Most of us have trained ourselves to avoid feeling anything for too much time. Some of us have come to rely on substances for that purpose. Let's change that by taking a few baby steps. If you suffer from anxiety, go into a room alone and experiment with how long you can sit in your anxiety before it becomes overwhelming. Time yourself. When you are done, go walk for ten minutes. How long were you able to tolerate your anxiety? One minute? Ten minutes? Thirty minutes? Were you able to sit in the discomfort for longer than you thought? Carpe diem, folks! You are stronger than you think. Over time, you may notice you have more ability to sit in discomfort than you think.

Let Go of "Normal"

In our work with veterans in various capacities, almost all of them have shared the same goal. Veterans want to feel level-headed and effective. They want to feel good again. They tell us they want to "feel normal." Some believe that using mood-altering substances can help them achieve this feeling.

What does "normal" mean? When we have an idea about what our experience needs to look like, we're probably trying to recapture a specific feeling, memory, or thought. You probably know someone who focuses on the past and even says things like "I wish it was like it used to be." Perhaps that person is you. It is natural to want to relive a previously enjoyed feeling or memory. But how much energy are you putting into trying to restore a past that is just that: the past?

It is healthier to view our past as something that informs our present and creates opportunities for our future. Let's take a moment to consider whether we may be using substances such as alcohol, drugs, or prescription medication in an effort to avoid the present in favor of a remembered feeling we've decided is "normal." Yes, we all want to feel good again, but trying to go back to what was in the past is not the answer. If we continue to seek a previous, idealized sense of how we used to feel (or look, or act), we also run the risk of losing what could be a new, realistic, and healthier normal.

What you thought was normal before the military, before your trauma, before your pain is not a goal to strive for now in your current life. Instead, take a step toward recalibrating what normal means, looks like, and feels like, and have the courage to make this change.

Create a new normal that reflects and embraces who you are now.

If you drew a picture of what your new normal looks and feels like, what would it show? Be realistic. Your recalibrated self may include your current pain, but along with these ongoing parts of your life, what tools, relationships, and attitudes have become a part of your new normal? Do you see how substances or other addictive behaviors may be holding you back from creating this new normal?

Let Go of Stigma

Many veterans worry that having problems with substance use or having mental health issues means they've done something wrong or that they're a bad or worthless person. They know that people who have addiction and mental health issues continue to be stigmatized in many circles, and so they're afraid to talk because they fear what others will think of them. *Will they think I'm weak? Will they be afraid of me? Will they think less of me or respect me less?* We sometimes assume we will be judged for how we're feeling or what we're thinking, and these internal questions are all the fuel we need to keep us from sharing a damn word.

But play it out in your mind the other way. What happens after we ask for help or express how we feel? What happens when a person listens to us, supports us, and acknowledges our pain? Does that stigma go away? The answer is quite simple: *It does if we let it.*

Earlier, we talked about changing our narrative by changing the way we frame or describe our story. One way we can change our story is by bringing new information, new people, and new events into it. Let's do a quick experiment. Imagine that a veteran buddy reaches out to you for support. He has been scared you'll judge him or think less of him if he admits being depressed, but he takes the risk now and opens up.

How do you respond?

There is a good chance you will tell him that his fears were nuts. You actually think more of him for having the courage to admit what he's facing, not less.

Let's apply that same logic to you. What will it take for you to trust that asking for help takes strength? Where did asking for help become stigmatizing for you? Does the stigma you place on yourself apply to others?

Take pride in getting help. It actually makes you more badass!

Many in the addiction recovery community have found that the moment someone realizes they are powerless over their drug of choice, they experience a sense of overwhelming relief. There is power in telling the truth and acknowledging a problem exists. There is power in admitting we were wrong or made a mistake. There is power in asking for help. Once we identify and admit we have a problem, we can do something to solve it.

If you have endured mental health issues or struggled to control your substance use, you are already badass in our book. You have struggled, persevered, and survived to keep going in your life. You've done whatever you can. That takes courage. You have tried to reduce the weight of your pain—weight that sits heavy on you and your family. That takes courage.

You picked up this book because you want to feel understood and you want to change your life. You want to end the covert mission of enduring pain and addiction all by yourself. It takes a badass person to do that! Self-reflection is the truest form of growth for an individual, and you are taking that step right now.

CHAPTER SEVEN

———

Pain and Trauma before
and after the Military

> *Oddly enough, I feel as if the abuse that I went through as a*
> *child helped me get through the first few years of being in the*
> *military. Having drill sergeants yell at me didn't really affect*
> *me the way it did other soldiers, because in the back of my*
> *mind I knew they wouldn't hit me like my father did. I instinc-*
> *tively followed orders and was proactive in accomplishing tasks*
> *and my assigned duties. In the back of my mind, I think I did*
> *these things so that I wouldn't get yelled at the way my father*
> *yelled at me for messing up.*
>
> **—JIM, US ARMY**

A NUMBER OF VETERANS volunteered to share their stories and experiences with us for this book. We're grateful for their trust and for their commitment to helping veterans like you feel more connected and less alone. Some of their stories were hard to hear— especially when veterans spoke about their childhoods and how they learned to understand and deal with physical, emotional, and social pain while growing up. Like Jim, who provided the quotation that starts this chapter, some described physical or emotional abuse. Others shared about growing up without money or the support of family. Many of the veterans talked about how and when they first started experimenting with alcohol or when they began using other substances to cope with the pain that was part of their pre-military lives.

Some veterans looked at these early experiences and situations as what "got them ready" for what they expected or anticipated the military life would be like. Veterans told us things like, "If I could deal with that, then maybe the Army wasn't going to be so bad," or, "I was used to getting yelled at, so why not become a marine?" Some of these veterans described joining the military as a kind of coping strategy. Becoming a soldier or sailor or marine or airman offered them an opportunity to resolve, escape, or move beyond the physical, emotional, or social pains that were part of their childhoods and start living a better life.

A few of the veterans saw the difficulties and lessons of their lives as evidence that they could endure and survive traumatic situations. This is sad, of course; kids shouldn't have to suffer abuse to grow up strong and healthy. Trauma is dangerous and destructive. However, these veterans' experiences also point to the truth that overcoming adversity can help build resilience—a trait that often leads to success and growth through challenges. We're still learning about how people develop resilience.

Asking veterans about their experiences with pain and trauma prior to the military helped us understand what contributed to or limited what was in their pain management toolboxes. We miss important information that could be key in helping veterans if we assume that everything we need to know about them and their experience starts with the day they entered the military. It's like looking at a photograph with the corner pieces torn off. You can try to guess what may have been there, but you'll never really get the whole picture.

This chapter helps complete the pain management picture we've been building together. We'll focus first on the experiences of, and ideas about, pain that you brought with you into the military. Next, we'll discuss how the pain management gear you were issued or picked up in childhood combines with what you learned and did as a member of the military. Finally, we'll look at how pain and trauma that persist after the military keep affecting your life as a veteran and what you can do to resolve, heal, or change the way you carry them.

Pain and addiction don't happen in a vacuum. Everything has an impact on everything else. Your problems with pain and/or addiction are not just happening by themselves. Exploring the interconnections between different chapters in your life story will help you consider how your experiences combine to impact your present issues with physical, emotional, and social pain. This type of life review can also help you assess the quality and usefulness of your coping gear.

Key topics in this chapter are childhood trauma and painful or traumatic experiences and events that happen after your time in the military. As usual, we'll close the chapter with a challenge to set down the gear that no longer works and pick up some new tools for healing and dealing with your pain. Tangible Next Steps will help you try out this new gear right away.

Adverse Childhood Experiences

Research on the effects of negative childhood experiences (called adverse childhood experiences, or ACEs) has found that family traumas like Jim describes above are more common than most people assume.[1] An "adverse childhood experience" is defined as an experience of physical, sexual, or emotional abuse; physical or emotional neglect; or any of a group of "household challenges" such as violence or mental illness in the household, parents' divorce or separation, chronic or infectious disease in the family, incarceration of a family member, or substance use issues. A majority of veterans have likely experienced a traumatic event before they ever enlisted in the military.[2]

One large study in the 1990s found that around two-thirds of the 17,000 participants reported having experienced at least one ACE before they turned eighteen.[3] Further research tells us that people who have experienced one or more ACEs in their childhood have increased risks for problems later in life—including problems with physical and mental health, the ability to function in relationships, or even the ability to hold jobs. ACEs predict decreased engagement in education, fewer employment opportunities, and a higher likelihood that we'll take risks with alcohol, drugs, and sex. ACEs are also cumulative, which means the more of these experiences we have in our history, the higher our risk for all these negative outcomes and ongoing problems.

The ACE research confirms what we've been saying throughout this book. Adding pain to pain and trauma to trauma compounds the physical, emotional, and social pain that many veterans endure. These previous experiences cannot be ignored. They likely impacted your time in the military, for better or for worse, and they continue to impact your daily functioning and quality of life now, especially if you have not worked through them. This is all the more reason to find effective, sustainable, and healthy ways to manage the pain and addiction, as well as resolve the trauma you've been carrying!

Trauma Stays with Us

Whether you think what you endured prior to joining the military ultimately helped or hurt you, that part of your life doesn't live in a separate box from everything else you've experienced. Childhood experiences have made you who you are. They affected how you handled yourself while in the military, and they're still part of your perception and personality now. Although we like to think we can compartmentalize our experiences, that's not how human beings work.

Keeping all the parts of our lives separate is quite literally impossible. Even years after an event happened, memories of what someone said or what you saw can affect you. You may still feel the impact that a car accident had on your hips and shoulder, or how your father broke your nose—which made it look the way it does now. Images, sounds, and smells can stay deep in the mind, even when we're not aware of those memories. Our bodies and minds carry scars and aches and reminders of everything that has happened to us.

Back in chapter 3, on physical pain, we described the way trauma does its damage. We used the image of a paper towel repeatedly getting wet and drying up again, making it less able to stay strong and flexible. Repeated floods of traumatic experiences and memories take the same kind of toll on our bodies and minds. If we don't work through our trauma, it can make us physically weaker and more exhausted. As we noted with ACEs, this can also harm our ability to deal with everyday situations and challenges.

Whether it's from a recent physical injury or a decades-old emotional wound, trauma affects both our mental and physical well-being. When these parts of us suffer, so do our relationships and our ability to navigate social settings or be comfortable around other people. Trauma can affect our ability to trust others and even how we present ourselves.

CHECKPOINT:

- How have you dealt with any trauma you experienced prior to joining the military?
- Did your experience of military service help you deal with your childhood pain? If so, how?
- Did your military experience make your prior pain or trauma worse? If so, how?

Pain, Trauma, and Addiction after the Military

—

You may be wondering why we've included a section on dealing with trauma, addiction, or pain after the military. This has been our subject throughout this book—haven't we covered everything by now? Hear us out for a little while longer.

Even though we've made a point of discussing how the gear you use to deal with pain is often influenced by the military culture and the expectations you embraced as a soldier, we want you to be careful **not to assume** that all trauma, pain, or problems with substances have roots in your time in the military. It's important that you remember that pain—and learning how to respond to and manage it—is an experience often shared by others. Veterans can also experience these issues regardless of the impact of their military service. We will provide more examples of this below.

Physical Pain Is Normal

Not all the aches and pains that veterans deal with are a direct result of their military experience. Life keeps happening. Physical pain that does not come from military trauma may include job-related injuries or chronic health conditions such as cancer, Parkinson's disease, or congestive heart failure. Other events that can impact a veteran's life include physical injuries from accidents, overexertion, or aging.

Some veterans have a difficult time accepting or tolerating these situations. Some feel annoyed or cheated, believing that they shouldn't have to experience life events that decrease their functioning and negatively affect their well-being. Although most of us won't admit it, some veterans feel like they've earned immunity from the things civilians suffer from or that their service should exempt them from "normal" physical maladies like heart disease or arthritis. Some may even feel shame that their newly acquired physical pain is not a direct result of their time in the military.

Others feel as though they should be strong enough to resist or ignore "normal" types of physical suffering.

Veterans can say things like "I was a Navy Seal or Army Ranger—how in the hell did I survive all of that but now I'm suffering from a back injury I got from gardening?" We know exactly how: our bodies change over time. For people who continue to imagine themselves as twenty-two-year-old marines who are in the best shape of their lives, this can be a hard reality to accept. Age alone makes us more susceptible to injuries and less able to bounce back like we once did. Recognizing these facts, grieving them, accepting them, and then letting them go is part of the challenge of living in the present.

Emotional Pain Is Normal

Dealing with emotional pain that is not directly connected to their military service can be very tough for some veterans. Many of us have a deep emotional connection to our military experiences, especially if we endured the trauma of combat losses or the death of a fellow veteran to suicide. In addition to continuing to carry these emotionally charged experiences, we can have a hard time setting down the emotional coping gear we once relied on to get us through when we were in the military.

Learning to interpret and respond to emotionally intense situations that happen outside the military takes recalibration of our coping mechanisms. Losing your father to Alzheimer's disease, for example, or finding out one of your children has been abused or bullied at school are situations that can elicit emotional responses, but neither demands a *military-style* emotional response. Veterans need to develop a new kind of situational awareness to help them recognize and deal with the normal emotional discomfort that comes with everyday life.

Developing this awareness starts with some self-assessment. Review the sections about survival mode in chapters 3 and 5. When you can assure yourself that your survival is not at stake in the current situation—even if it feels emotionally uncomfortable—then you can dial back the amount of emotional energy you're expending and dial up your thoughtfulness and problem-solving skills.

Social Pain Is Normal

As veterans return to civilian life, many experience the sense that other people don't quite understand what they've been through. Relearning how to lean on and communicate with loved ones at home about how to handle these situations is vital. This can also be difficult and frustrating to do.

If you're a veteran who laments that people don't know or appreciate what you experienced while serving, let's flip this idea on its head. Take a moment to consider that the people you left behind when you entered the military have lived lives and had experiences that you haven't witnessed or participated in either. In a very real way, you don't understand what they have been through.

Many veterans return to emotionally difficult family relationships after serving. If your spouse cheated on you while you were overseas or your child has been struggling academically or socially in your absence, you may feel guilty for not having been there for them or angry and hurt about being betrayed or let down. This is extremely difficult for some veterans. They may come home to expectations that they need to "fix" what happened while they were gone or that they should step up and take responsibility.

Please know many of these issues have most likely developed over time, and you are not responsible for immediately addressing or solving everything just because you are home now. You are responsible for how *you* show up and what *you* choose to do. Close family relationships, and developments in those relationships, take time and patience. Offer yourself some of that patience as well.

We can tell ourselves things like *If I were here and not serving, maybe this wouldn't have happened* or *I hate what was taken from me because of my time away.* We may also hear similar messages from our loved ones. Statements like "If you had been here, maybe things would be different" or "Do you know how much your not being here has impacted us?" can be difficult to deal with. A sense of guilt, shame, or regret can drive a wedge between veterans and their loved ones. These feelings can also make us doubt the value of our time in the military.

Learning to manage your own emotional pain responses will help you navigate these challenges. You can practice this with friends or with a therapist. Start by getting used to discussing or sharing emotional experiences with lower stakes and expressing feelings that don't seem overwhelming. As you get more comfortable addressing less complicated emotional issues with people you trust, you'll be better able to handle harder conversations with loved ones where trust comes less easily.

Other socially painful experiences include trying to develop new friendships with coworkers or neighbors, navigating college or some other educational environment, or settling into a job that is run very differently than the ship, tank, or aircraft you worked on. It's natural to compare these social settings to your military experience.

It may help to know that these feelings are not unique to you. Everyone has felt out of place. Taking on new experiences and entering unknown social settings is part of normal life, even if these situations feel lonely or frustrating. Rely on your strengths and your history of overcoming challenges to meet these opportunities. Remember to use the tools we shared with you in the social pain chapter. Work on adjusting your expectations and assumptions. Keep in mind that comparisons often lead to disappointment, and remember that you can manage your expectations for yourself and others. You survived basic. You can do this.

The Disease of Addiction Is Normal

We've noted that substance use and addiction are common among veterans. We've also discussed some of the reasons that service members and veterans use addictive substances and behaviors to cope with or avoid their pain. If, during your time in the military, you experienced significant life stressors, trauma, and/or pain, you may be at a higher risk for addiction. This fact leads some veterans to blame their time in the military for their substance use disorder. This is not always the main reason, however. Remember that there are many factors that can increase the risk for addiction, including things we experienced before the military and our genetics. Our life experiences after we get out can play a role as well.

We need to make a distinction between the ongoing challenges veterans face from their time in the military and the things that can happen to all of us—veteran and civilian alike—simply because we're human. Some of the physical, emotional, and social pain you experience as a veteran may not be directly connected to your military experience at all.

People can and do become addicted to substances for many reasons. Work-related injuries, for example, lead many people to begin taking prescription opioids to manage their physical pain. Too often this turns into a source of daily comfort and the use becomes problematic. Others use substances to numb painful or overwhelming emotional experiences like divorces, job losses, or the deaths of family members. On the social side, sometimes fitting in with a new work or friend group means going for drinks every day. Eventually you may come to realize this is spinning out of control. Even if you didn't experience problems with substances in the military, that may change in the years following your service.

At any time in our lives, we may experience major difficulties that will require us to endure, manage, or cope with pain. The question is not *whether* we'll need to cope, it's *how* we will choose to do so. If you rely on alcohol, other drugs, or addictive behaviors as coping gear, you're increasing your risk of developing an addiction—a disorder that leads to other kinds of physical, emotional, and social problems and pain. Throughout this book, we have provided Tangible Next Steps to help you develop healthier tools to deal with pain. We hope you've found gear that fits and strategies that make sense for you.

Tangible Next Steps

—

Review Your Life before and after the Military

Did you experience issues with substances, trauma, or pain prior to your time in the military? How about after? Here's an exercise that will help you take an inventory of these experiences and how you handled them.

Get a piece of paper, a notebook, or your phone and make some lists. You'll want to have four columns or four lists. Label the first column "Significant Life Events." Beneath that heading write as many *significant* events as you can think of from your life before and after the military. You decide what counts as significant. Put a "B" next to the events that happened before your military service and an "A" beside events that happened after. You might also decide to include events during the military. This is up to you!

How did you handle the events you listed? Did you bottle up your emotions, turn to drugs or alcohol, get in fights, or something else? Maybe your responses included healthy strategies like getting help. Label the second column "How I Handled It." Beside each significant event, make a quick note about how you responded. This can include how you felt. It should also briefly describe what you did to cope with those events when they occurred.

Label the third column "What I Could Have Done Differently." Write a few notes in this column that describe other, healthier ways you might have handled or responded to your significant life events. Even when we managed our significant life event well, we can learn and improve for the future, so jot down ways that you could have responded even better than you did.

Finally, make a fourth column under the heading "What I Will Do Differently." Make notes here about how you will cope with or handle similar circumstances or situations when and if they happen again in the future. Focus on what you will *do*. Again, this is where you can use tools from this book.

Here are a few ideas from this book to get you started. What other coping strategies can you try?

- "Right-size" my expectations.
- Avoid assumptions.
- Let go of comparisons.
- Ask clarifying questions.
- Reach out to a friend or loved one.
- Conserve my energy.
- Breathe.
- Relax my body.
- Tune in to what my senses are telling me.

- Enlist professional help.
- Pay attention to my body's signals.
- Seek connection by being curious about the other person.
- Keep caring.
- Allow space for grief.
- Accept.
- Adjust.

Remember, Pain and Addiction Do NOT Exist in a Vacuum

Most likely your pain and/or addiction problems are not just happening by themselves. Explore the interconnections between your various life experiences, even the experiences outside of the military, and their impact on you. Explore how things affect each other. Remember what we have talked about: physical pain impacts both emotional and social pain and vice versa. With how complicated this is, also remember this internal pep talk: you are not responsible for fixing everything.

CHAPTER EIGHT

—

The New Mission

> *The hardest part of leaving the military is not being told what to do. We become so conditioned to having a superior to instruct us, so it is difficult to manage our own lives when we have been reliant upon others to do it. Falling in line is easy for us, but making our own line is tough.*
>
> —CHRIS, US AIR FORCE

> *I personally took forever to open up about my mental health. Now I do whatever I can to get others to open up. My advice: be patient with us, we aren't used to being listened to. We spent years being told what to do and what not to do, like not going to sick call or be seen for injuries, physical or mental, because we would be seen as a "shit bag" soldier. Be patient with us is all I ask.*
>
> —KYLE, US ARMY

> *Most vets understand this, but it is very hard for us to drop the facade and ask for help.*
>
> —EMILY, US COAST GUARD

IMAGINE ONE NIGHT you are called to the hospital. Your grandfather, a World War II veteran, has been ill. The cancer that's dogged him for decades is finally taking him. You're told he may not last the night. You've always admired your grandfather. He had grit and determination, and he was the strongest person you knew, even though he walked for more than half his life with a limp from a war injury.

As you enter the hospital room, you look down at the bed and see your grandfather lying there, frail and small. He notices you and his eyes brighten. Struggling to breathe, he motions for you to come closer. As you lean down beside his face, you see two tears trickle slowly down his cheek.

You have never seen your grandfather cry, not even once. You wonder what he's about to say. This is the same man who never talked about his pain, never talked about the war he fought in, never complained about anything in his life. As you draw even closer, he whispers something. It sounds like he is saying, "Sorry, I am so sorry." You ask him, "What you are sorry about?"

Over the next few minutes, your grandfather opens up. With a raspy voice, he tells you the story of a specific experience that happened during the war—a traumatic memory that has haunted him for his whole life. It seems he needed to get this out of his head before he died, and he chose you as the person to help him hold the memory one last time. Moments later, he passes away. Now fighting your own tears as you sit beside his body, you wonder what made him keep this story from you.

Many people hold on to pain their entire life. They may be afraid to tell others. They may think no one will understand. Maybe they don't want to admit they need help or don't know where to find help. Veterans may have all kinds of reasons for keeping silent about the pain they experience and the burdens they carry. You have your own explanations for what has made you do what you've done, and how your own experiences helped or harmed you.

Our experience as psychologists and health care providers has taught us a few important things about pain. We know that everybody has a desire to free themselves from pain. We know that people could use some help learning how to do that. We also know that many veterans use means such as alcohol, other drugs, or sex to stop feeling pain or try to make it hurt less. Yet it returns.

We do not want you to live your entire life alone with pain that could instead be shared, processed, taken away, lessened, or relieved. By reading this book, you're already following your desire to feel better, to be understood, and to learn healthier and more sustainable ways to deal with your pain. You are reaching for help and taking a step toward less pain and more joy. You're ending the covert mission you've been on. You're joining a growing force of veterans who rely on each other and the circles of support around you to share your stories, set down burdens, and heal. You're on a new mission. This is worth celebrating.

It's also worth pursuing, so keep going.

Keep Going

——

Throughout this book, we've shared stories and experiences of fellow veterans who have gone through many of the same things you have. Many are still working through their pain and dealing with addiction. Their stories demonstrate that achieving a healthier veteran life is a cadence march, not a sprint. You're on the same march—the same mission of finding relief from physical, emotional, and social pain.

As you pursue this mission, we want you to have the best and most up-to-date gear possible. We want you to use this gear to keep going, to keep taking steps toward a better way of living with and managing your pain and fighting enemies like addiction, isolation, and despair.

Tangible Next Steps have been an important part of this book. In this final chapter, we're offering one last list—consider it the "best of" compilation. Here are five things you should remember even if everything else we've written fades away.

1. Own Your Pain, Own Your Addiction

Ending your covert mission means you aren't going to hide or dismiss your pain and/or addiction any longer. Keeping these things inside allows them to grow bigger and worse. As they do, they'll control more of your life than they do now. It's time to own the pain you're experiencing. If you're also turning to substance use or relying on some other addictive behavior to numb or forget your pain, it's time to own the possibility of addiction and get help for it.

You didn't ask for these things to happen to you, but since they have, they're your responsibility to address. This is a mind shift step, and you're the only one who can take it. When you're able to claim ownership of the painful parts of your experience before, during, and after your military service, you have taken the first step toward healing that pain.

Owning your physical pain may lead you to decide that it's finally time to seek services like working with a pain provider, going to a physical therapist, or getting surgery. Owning your emotional pain means embracing the truth that difficult feelings and emotions can be as painful as physical injuries. Owning social pain will help you recognize that relationships are rewarding and valuable, and that they can help you grow and be happy even when they're hard or need healing. Owning your experience of addiction—or your concern about your substance use—may allow you to open up to someone who can connect you with a treatment program or peer support group like AA or NA.

Owning the ways all these pains affect each other can help you notice when that's happening and take action to make your situation better. That's the whole point of this book! Once we take responsibility for our pain and addiction, we can take action to start changing our experience. As we do, we'll see our lives improve.

2. Relax

At the end of the day, one key piece of gear for finding relief from any kind of pain is relaxation. Pain of any sort is exhausting, and if we're going to deal with it well, we need to rest. Finding reliable ways to calm our bodies and minds provides physical relief for our spinal cords and causes the pain and trauma response mechanisms in our bodies to stand down.

Relaxation techniques will help you deal with impulsive moments too. When you feel like nothing else may work against your pain besides taking a drink or using other substances, well-practiced relaxation exercises like meditation or deep breathing can save you from bad decisions and worse outcomes. Relaxation is free, always available, and the most effective pain-relief process in the world.

3. Reflect

Reflection simply means paying attention to yourself and what's happening around you while connecting to what's happening inside you. As we have discussed, this helps grow awareness. Taking time to think through the various kinds of pain you're facing can help you develop perspective and see possibilities. Reflection allows you to consider how painful events and situations in your life may be impacting your feelings, relationships, and physical functioning.

This can feel like a hard or time-consuming task. It doesn't have to be. You don't have to sit and think for hours and hours. Instead, you can find time for reflection while you shovel snow or when you go for a walk on a summer evening. You can reflect while driving or when you stand at the sink washing dishes. Some veterans keep journals or write letters to help them process or reflect. Some find a trusted person like a counselor or close friend to do this with.

Take time to reflect on the good things in your life as well as the harder and more challenging parts. The idea is that by listening to your thoughts and paying attention to the feelings in your body, you get to know yourself better. Unlike just stewing on or fuming about things that aren't going well in your life, reflection provides you with information about yourself. Other reflection activities like painting, drawing, or woodworking can help you organize or process thoughts and feelings in a more creative way. You have to find what works best for you. Sometimes simply getting these things out of our heads lightens our load and provides relief. Reflection can reveal new insights and ideas. You can use this information to make choices and do things that will help you feel better.

4. Dammit, Just Talk!

This one speaks for itself (see what we did there?).

By the time you've reached this point in the book, you have heard the invitation to open up more than once. This is the step that truly represents the end of the covert mission of coping with pain and addiction. Talking with another person about your pain or addiction starts the shared mission of finding relief. When you open your mouth, you're also opening up a new kind of future.

Trust that your voice is worth listening to. What you have to say is important. Whenever you share with others, you open yourself to the possibility of learning from their experience and perspective. Sharing in this way can help you feel more connected and better respected. It can help make your pain burden feel less heavy and more bearable, because you're no longer carrying it alone.

Sharing heavy stuff can make you feel vulnerable. It can feel like you're in unknown territory. Take your time when you're deciding whom you will share with and what you will ask of the person you select. Maybe you'll choose to try it out by sharing something minor from your life and then reflect on how you felt before moving on to sharing harder experiences and feelings. Know and trust that talking is beneficial. Sharing our thoughts and feelings, as well as our hopes and fears, connects us to the people we care about. It also allows us to be seen and validated and cared for by people who can help us. This includes family, friends, significant others, other veterans, non-veterans, and health care providers.

5. Use Your Veteran Voice to Help Others

We asked the veterans who added their voices to this book to answer ten questions. Then we used their answers for the quotations that start each chapter and other quotes throughout the book. These veterans wanted their stories and statements to be part of our work because they wanted to help other veterans. This willingness to offer support and assistance to fellow veterans is a wonderful characteristic of the veteran community.

Your voice as a veteran is important too. We want you to be part of the movement that helps veterans end the covert mission of silent suffering and join the mission in which sharing pain and finding relief is a normal part of everyday life. You can start by exploring your own story and sharing it with someone else. If you'd like, you can use the same questions we asked the veterans who contributed to this book. They're listed below.

These questions are intended to help you explore and develop your thoughts around pain and addiction, especially as these things have been part of your life experience before, during, and after the military. You can write out your responses, or just spend some time thinking about them.

- Before entering the military, did you experience any adverse events, such as trauma? If so, what kind of impact did that have on your experience in the military, if any?

- How did you manage your emotions or feelings before entering the military? What messages/values were taught in the military culture?

- Please share your experience about using substances (e.g., alcohol, drugs) to cope with pain related to your military experience.

- Provide a few examples of emotional pain that you have experienced as a direct result of your military experience.

- Provide a few examples of physical pain that you have experienced as a direct result of your military experience.

- Provide a few examples of spiritual pain that you have experienced as a direct result of your military experience.

- Following your time in the military, how have you coped with your pain or mental health?

- What is your relationship with the veteran community? How do you connect with other veterans? What is it like to talk with other veterans about your experience in the military?

- What has been the hardest part of your transition out of the military?

- If there is one thing a mental health clinician should know about the veteran community, what would it be?

Developing your own veteran voice is a reflective activity. Responding to these questions may help you uncover some thoughts or feelings that you haven't considered before. Your answers might also reveal some things you'd like to explore more or some thoughts that you're ready to let go.

Your answers are for you. At some point you may decide to share them with somebody important to you, like a spouse or significant other, or a family member or close friend. You may choose to share them with a former battle buddy or another veteran. Your answers could also be part of a longer conversation with a therapist or counselor.

New Gear for a New Time

Throughout this book, we've made the case that it's time to drop your rucksack full of old gear. Some of the pain management tools and coping strategies you used in childhood or during your time in the military need to be retired. We want to honor the fact that these things have served you, even if they came with some downsides and caused pain of their own. You used the gear you had and did your best with the tools at hand. And you survived every mission. You made it to where you are today.

Today is a new time for you, and you're faced with a new mission. You get to empty out that ruck, shake the dust and sand from it, and choose which tools go back in. You get to take the best of the lessons from your past and leave the rest behind.

We've offered a bunch of new pain and addiction management gear, and there's more out there. New gear being issued today includes various strategies for understanding how our thoughts affect our feelings and actions, techniques for calming the mind and body, reliable support systems, therapies for reducing pain, treatments and support for recovering from addiction, and many more. These are just some of the brand spanking new and shiny tools you can learn to use to better deal with pain as you move forward in accomplishing the mission of your life.

Take this gear and keep going! You are already badass for reading this book. You've taken important steps in changing your relationship with pain. Now, armed with new gear, let's lock and load our new strategies, oil up the new tracks that will guide the vehicle of change, and start this convoy with confidence.

NOTES

Chapter Two

1. Karen O. Dunivin, "Military Culture: Change and Continuity," *Armed Forces & Society* 20, no. 4 (July 1994): 531–47; W. Arkin and L. R. Dobrofsky, "Military Socialization and Masculinity," *Journal of Social Issues* 34, no. 1 (1978): 151–68, https://doi.org/10.1111/j.1540-4560.1978.tb02546.x.
2. Dustin Brockberg, "Predicting VA Help-Seeking Decision-Making in OIF/OEF/OND Veterans: Examining the Role of Veteran Culture" (PhD diss., University of Wisconsin–Madison, 2019), 109–13.

Chapter Three

1. Centers for Disease Control and Prevention, "Drug Overdose Deaths Remain High," last reviewed June 2, 2022, https://www.cdc.gov/drugoverdose/deaths/index.html.
2. Centers for Disease Control and Prevention, "Drug Overdose Deaths in the U.S. Top 100,000 Annually," last reviewed November 17, 2021, https://www.cdc.gov/nchs/pressroom/nchs_press_releases/2021/20211117.htm.
3. U.S. Department of Veterans Affairs Office of Public and Intergovernmental Affairs, "VA Reduces Prescription Opioid Use by 64% during Past Eight Years," news release, July 30, 2020, https://www.va.gov/opa/pressrel/pressrelease.cfm?id=5492.
4. Ronald Melzack and Patrick D. Wall, "Pain Mechanisms: A New Theory: A Gate Control System Modulates Sensory Input from the Skin before It Evokes Pain Perception and Response," *Science* 150, no. 3699 (1965): 971–79.

Chapter Four

1. U.S. Department of Veterans Affairs Office of Mental Health and Suicide Prevention, "2021 National Veteran Suicide Prevention Annual Report" (September 2021), https://www.mentalhealth.va.gov/docs/data-sheets/2021/2021-National-Veteran-Suicide-Prevention-Annual-Report-FINAL-9-8-21.pdf.
2. U.S. Department of Commerce, U.S. Census Bureau, "Those Who Served: America's Veterans from World War II to the War on Terror: American Community Survey Report," June 2020, https://www.census.gov/content/dam/Census/library/publications/2020/demo/acs-43.pdf.

Chapter Six

1. Jenni B. Teeters, Cynthia L. Lancaster, Delisa G. Brown, and Sudie E. Back, "Substance Use Disorders in Military Veterans: Prevalence and Treatment Challenges," *Substance Abuse and Rehabilitation* 8 (August 2017): 69–77, https://doi.org/10.2147/SAR.S116720.
2. Teeters et al., "Substance Use Disorders in Military Veterans," 69–77.
3. Tim O'Brien, *The Things They Carried: A Work of Fiction* (Boston: Houghton Mifflin Harcourt, 2010).
4. U.S. Department of Veterans Affairs, "Substance Use," accessed May 2022, https://www.mentalhealth.va.gov/substance-use/index.asp.

Chapter Seven

1. Centers for Disease Control and Prevention, "Fast Facts: Preventing Adverse Childhood Experiences," last reviewed April 6, 2022, https://www.cdc.gov/violenceprevention/aces/fastfact.html.
2. U.S. Department of Veterans Affairs, Veterans Health Administration, "From Science to Practice: Premilitary Risk Factors Associated with Suicide among Veterans," March 2019, https://www.mentalhealth.va.gov/suicide_prevention/docs/Literature-Review-Premilitary-Trauma-CLEARED-3-5-19.pdf.
3. Vincent J. Felitti, Robert F. Anda, Dale Nordenberg, David F. Williamson, Alison M. Spitz, Valerie Edwards, Mary P. Koss, and James S. Marks, "Relationship of Childhood Abuse and Household Dysfunction to Many of the Leading Causes of Death in Adults: The Adverse Childhood Experiences (ACE) Study," *American Journal of Preventive Medicine* 14, no. 4 (May 1998): 245–58, https://doi.org/10.1016/S0749-3797(98)00017-8.

ABOUT THE AUTHORS

Dustin Brockberg, PhD, is a licensed psychologist working in the field of substance use and co-occurring disorders. He served in the United States Army from 2004 to 2008, including a deployment to Iraq. His clinical interests include veteran-related issues, grief, loss, affect phobia, and trauma.

Kerry Brockberg, PhD, is a licensed psychologist working in the field of rehabilitation. Her current practice focuses on individuals with chronic pain, brain injury, and other chronic illnesses and disabilities. She specializes in the development of tangible, psychological approaches connecting the mind and body in better understanding overall functioning and quality of life.

ABOUT HAZELDEN PUBLISHING

As part of the Hazelden Betty Ford Foundation, Hazelden Publishing offers both cutting-edge educational resources and inspirational books. Our print and digital works help guide individuals in treatment and recovery, as well as their loved ones.

Professionals who work to prevent and treat addiction also turn to Hazelden Publishing for evidence-based curricula, digital content solutions, and videos for use in schools, treatment and correctional programs, and community settings. We also offer training for implementation of our curricula.

Through published and digital works, Hazelden Publishing extends the reach of healing and hope to individuals, families, and communities affected by addiction and related issues.

For information about Hazelden publications,
please call **800-328-9000**
or visit us online at **hazelden.org/bookstore**.